Pediatric Type II Diabetes

Pediatric Type II Diabetes

GRACE KIM, MD
Assistant Professor
Endocrine
Seattle Childrens Hospital
Seattle, WA, United States

ELSEVIER

ELSEVIER

3251 Riverport Lane
St. Louis, Missouri 63043

Publisher: Mica Haley
Acquisition Editor: Nancy Duffy
Editorial Project Manager: Jennifer Horigan
Production Project Manager: Kiruthika Govindaraju
Cover Designer: Alan Studholme

Typeset by TNQ Technologies

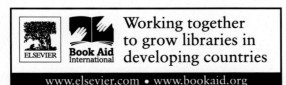

List of Contributors

Ram Weiss, MD, PhD
Department of Pediatrics
Ruth Rappaport Children's Hospital, Rambam
    Medical Center, Haifa, Israel

Allison S. LaRoche, MD, MPH
Pediatric Endocrinology Fellow
Pediatric Endocrinology
University of Washington
Seattle, WA, United States

Grace Kim, MD
Assistant Professor
Endocrine
Seattle Childrens Hospital
Seattle, WA, United States

Camille Michaud, MD
Attending Physician
Pediatric Endocrinology
The Children's Hospital of Philadelphia
Philadelphia, PA, United States

Assistance Professor of Pediatrics
Perelman School of Medicine
University of Pennsylvania
Philadelphia, PA, United States

Rochelle Naylor, MD
Instructor
Section of Adult and Pediatric Endocrinology,
    Diabetes & Metabolism
University of Chicago
Chicago, IL, United States

Louis Philipson, MD, PhD
Professor
Medicine and Pediatrics
University of Chicago
Chicago, IL, United States

Susan Tucker, MD
Fellow, Pediatric Endocrinology
Section of Adult and Pediatric Endocrinology,
    Diabetes, and Metabolism
The University of Chicago
Chicago, IL, United States

Lynne L. Levitsky, MD
Department of Pediatrics
Massachusetts General Hospital
Boston, MA, United States

Charumathi Baskaran, MD
MD
Endocrinology
Boston Children's Hospital
Boston, MA, United States

Lorraine Katz, MD
Professor of Pediatrics
Division of Endocrinology
Children's Hospital of Philadelphia
Perelman School of Medicine
University of Pennsylvania
Philadelphia, PA, United States

Ryan Farrell, MD
Assistant Professor
Pediatrics
Rainbow Babies and Children's Hospital
Cleveland, OH, United States

Shakira F. Suglia, ScD, MS
Associate Professor
Epidemiology
Emory University
Atlanta, GA, United States

Heba M. Ismail, MBBCH, MSC, PhD
Assistant Professor
Pediatric Endocrinology
Children's Hospital of Pittsburgh of UPMC
Pittsburgh, PA, United States

Marissa Avolio, MD
Fellow
Pediatric Endocrinology
Children's Hospital of Pittsburgh of UPMC
Pittsburgh, PA, United States

Nicola Santoro, MD, PhD
Associate Research Scientist
Pediatrics
Yale University School of Medicine
New Haven, CT, United States

Michelle A. Van Name, MD
Assistant Professor
Pediatrics
Yale School of Medicine
New Haven, CT, United States

Amy S. Shah, MD, MS
Associate Professor
Pediatrics
Cincinnati Children's Hospital Medical Center
Cincinnati, OH, United States

Professor
Surgery
Children's Hospital Colorado
Aurora, CO, United States

Thomas Inge, MD, PhD
Professor and Division Chief
Pediatric Surgery
Children's Hospital Colorado
Aurora, CO, United States

Erin Richardson, MD
Rainbow Babies and Children's Hospital
University Hospitals Cleveland Medical Center
Cleveland, OH, United States

Alfonso Galderisi, MD
Pediatrics Endocrinology
Yale School of Medicine
New Haven, CT, United States

Mariangela Martino, MD
Department of Pediatrics
Yale University School of Medicine
New Haven, CT, United States

Brett Barrett, DO, MS
Pediatric Endocrinology - The Children's Hospital of
    Philadelphia
Philadelphia, PA, United States

Aim of Pediatric Type II Diabetes

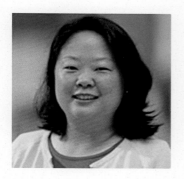

The aim of *Pediatric Type II Diabetes* is to provide concise information on the diagnosis, treatment, and complications of pediatric type II diabetes. The audience is pediatricians, primary care physicians, and pediatric endocrinologists. I believe we have assembled a book on comprehensive topics relating to type II diabetes.

Grace Kim, MD
Assistant Professor
Endocrine
Seattle Childrens Hospital
Seattle, WA, United States

Contents

CHAPTER 1

Pathophysiology of Insulin Resistance and Type 2 Diabetes

RAM WEISS, MD, PHD

Type 2 diabetes (T2DM) is a recent addition to the medical conditions encountered in the pediatric age group. Prior to the 1980s, this condition was considered an "adult onset" disease and was rarely if at all diagnosed in childhood.[1] In the mid-1990s, first descriptions of T2DM in adolescents appeared and in parallel with the rising prevalence of obesity, this disease is now encountered more commonly in the pediatric age group.[2] The strong coincidental association with obesity stems from one of the key factors driving the development of T2DM—insulin resistance.[3] To develop T2DM, two defects must be present: insulin resistance and β-cell failure. Importantly, insulin resistance is a common trait in the general population as well as in obese children and adolescents.[4] Most insulin resistant individuals do not develop diabetes because their β-cells are able to compensate appropriately for the ambient resistance by secreting more insulin. Only failure to compensate appropriately (β-cell failure) will result initially in altered glucose metabolism (a group of conditions called "prediabetes") and may eventually progress to overt T2DM.

PATHOPHYSIOLOGY OF INSULIN RESISTANCE

Insulin resistance is a term used to describe a relative reduction in the metabolic response to insulin within its target tissues that are involved in glucose metabolism. These target tissues include the liver (hepatic glucose production is crucial for the fasting state), muscle (skeletal muscle glucose uptake governs the postabsorptive state), the endocrine pancreas, and adipose tissue. In the fasting state, normoglycemia is maintained by production of glucose by the liver via glycogen breakdown and gluconeogenesis. Hepatic glucose production is regulated by two main mechanisms:

hormones secreted by the endocrine pancreas (glucagon and insulin) and by autonomic innervation.[5] The dominant hormone of the fasting state is glucagon that induces glycogenolysis and gluconeogenesis, as does the autonomic sympathetic arm.[6] Adipose tissue during fasting predominantly secretes free fatty acids (FFAs) produced via lipolysis to provide an alternative fuel to glucose while muscle takes up minimal glucose from the circulation. In the postabsorptive state dominated by insulin, hepatic glucose production is suppressed by insulin and the parasympathetic autonomic system while skeletal muscle glucose uptake is increased via trafficking of the glucose transporter 4 (GLUT-4) to the myocyte membrane. Adipose tissue in the postabsorptive state is characterized by enhanced lipogenesis. Importantly, the brain plays a dominant role in glucose metabolism via a mechanism called glucose effectiveness, which describes the effects of ambient glucose on its own uptake, independent of insulin.[7] Glucose effectiveness has a major impact on whole body glucose disposal in postabsorptive conditions (basal insulin concentrations) estimated at ~70%, while during exposure to typical postprandial insulin concentrations during a hyperinsulinemic-euglycemic clamp, the relative contribution of effectiveness to glucose disposal drops to ~30%. Following oral ingestion of a glucose load resulting in dynamic insulin concentrations, the relative effect of glucose effectiveness on whole body glucose disposal is estimated at 50%.[7]

All organs described above may demonstrate resistance to the effects of insulin to a certain degree. This resistance describes an inhibition of the signal transduction pathway that is involved in glucose metabolism (such as gluconeogenesis or glycogen metabolism) but not necessarily in other targets of insulin signal transduction such as lipid metabolism. Several mechanisms have been proposed to explain how this inhibition

Pediatric Type II Diabetes. https://doi.org/10.1016/B978-0-323-55138-0.00001-2.

occurs. The leading theory is that fatty acid derivates of intracellular lipid droplets inhibit critical elements of the insulin signal transduction pathway.[8] These derivates (mainly fatty acyl CoAs and ceramide) inhibit insulin signal transduction via activation of activation of a serine/threonine kinase cascade (possibly initiated by protein kinase Cθ), eventually leading to phosphorylation of serine/threonine sites on insulin receptor substrate 1 and 2. Serine-phosphorylated forms of IRS 1 and 2 fail to activate PI 3-kinase resulting in reduced activation of glucose transport in skeletal muscle or suppression of gluconeogenesis in the liver.[9]

It is well established that in the pediatric age group, obesity is the leading feature associated with reduced insulin sensitivity.[10] Importantly, not all obese children are insulin resistant.[11] Recent studies performed in obese children and adolescents have shown that the pattern of lipid partitioning and not the degree of obesity per se is the best correlate of insulin resistance.[12] Lipid partitioning describes a specific profile of lipid depot distribution characterized by the deposition of fat within the intraabdominal compartment (visceral fat) as well as within the liver and skeletal muscle. The ability of subcutaneous fat to store excess lipid is probably the determining factor in the development of insulin resistance.[13] Those able to store large amounts of fat in this depot and spare liver and muscle maintain relative insulin sensitivity while those that are unable to expand it tend to accumulate excess intraabdominal and liver/muscle fat. It has been shown that, in equally obese adolescents (by means of body mass index and percent body fat) who differ in their degree of insulin sensitivity, those who are more resistant are characterized by larger amounts of visceral, intrahepatic, and intramyocellular lipid.[14] This can be expressed in other terms as the ratio of visceral fat to total abdominal fat—where those with a larger ratio (who are not necessarily more obese) tend to be much more insulin resistant and have greater amounts of intrahepatic fat. Similar to muscle and liver, lipid deposition within the pancreas has been shown to associate with altered β-cell function,[15] yet whether it has a direct role in the pathophysiology of T2DM is controversial.[16] Moreover, lower suppression of c-peptide secretion has been demonstrated in obese insulin resistant adolescents during euglycemic-hyperinsulinemic clamps along with reduced suppression of glucagon.[17] Whether "islet insulin resistance" and α-cell upregulation are a result of intrapancreatic lipid deposition is still to be determined. The mechanism of glucose effectiveness governed by specific central nervous system nuclei has also been shown to be altered in obese children with greater waist circumference (a surrogate of intraabdominal lipid deposition) and thus is unable to compensate for the reduction of insulin-dependent glucose disposal typical of whole body insulin resistance.[18]

A third important contributor to the typical insulin resistant milieu observed in obese children is adipose tissue that also may manifest resistance to the effects of insulin. As insulin suppresses lipolysis and induces lipogenesis in adipose tissue, resistance to its effects results in a shift of this balance toward greater lipolysis resulting in enhanced secretion of free fatty acids to the circulation.[19] Obese insulin resistant adolescents showed reduced suppression of FFA secretion during oral glucose tolerance tests and increased concentrations of fasting FFAs.[20] In obese children with normal glucose tolerance, an increase in adipose tissue insulin resistance was related to an increase in 2-h glucose levels. A tight relationship exists between visceral fat as well as the visceral-to-subcutaneous fat ratio with the adipose tissue insulin resistance. It has been shown that acute exposure to FFAs during euglycemic-hyperinsulinemic clamps results in an acute reduction of whole body insulin sensitivity.[21] Thus, basal and postprandial exposure to greater concentrations of FFAs, as shown in obese insulin resistant children, may have a similar peripheral effect enhancing overall resistance to the effects of insulin on skeletal muscle.

An additional mechanism driving the development of resistance to the effects of insulin in liver, muscle, and adipose tissue is the presence of inflammatory mediators. Subcutaneous and visceral fat is typically infiltrated by cells of the immune system, mainly macrophages, which secrete typical chemokines and induce the typical low-grade inflammatory profile that is commonly observed in obese adolescents.[22] The innate immune cell sensor leucine-rich pyrin domain containing 3 (NLRP3) inflammosome is one of the factors implicated in adipose tissue inflammation and the pathogenesis of insulin resistance. Obese adolescents with a high visceral-to-subcutaneous fat ratio show greater infiltration of macrophages within the subcutaneous fat depot and higher expression of the NLRP3 inflammosome-related genes. The increase in these markers of inflammation is present in parallel with a decrease in the expression of genes related to insulin sensitivity and lipogenesis. In addition, the concentration of ceramide within subcutaneous fat correlates with the expression of multiple inflammosome-related genes.[23] The presence of subcutaneous fat depot infiltration by macrophages and other cells of the immune system and upregulation of the NLRP3 inflammosome along with increased systemic and intraadipose concentrations of ceramide may contribute to the limited expansion capability of subcutaneous abdominal adipose tissue leading to development of altered abdominal lipid partitioning and insulin resistance. In addition, macrophage infiltration into white adipose tissue induces increased lipolysis that further increases hepatic de novo triglyceride synthesis and hyperlipidemia due to increased fatty acid esterification.[9] Macrophage-induced adipose tissue lipolysis further stimulates hepatic gluconeogenesis, thus promoting hyperglycemia in both absorptive and postabsorptive states via increased fatty acid fluxes to the liver leading to increased hepatic acetyl-CoA that activates pyruvate carboxylase and thus induces increased glycerol conversion to glucose.[24] Thus, impaired insulin signaling in adipose tissue, caused by macrophage and other immune cell-induced inflammation, leads to a specific adverse substrate flux to the liver that results in accelerated intrahepatic lipid synthesis and thus to insulin resistance in the signal transduction pathway segment involved in suppression of gluconeogenesis.

Thus, insulin resistance in obese children is tightly linked to a typical lipid-partitioning pattern characterized by increased amounts of lipid within the main insulin-responsive tissues (skeletal muscle and liver) and a relatively reduced capacity to increase subcutaneous fat stores. Insulin resistance in the setting of childhood obesity thus results from a combination of altered functions of insulin-responsive target cells and the accumulation of macrophages that secrete proinflammatory mediators. Moreover, the adipose tissue of obese adolescents may also manifest insulin resistance resulting in lower suppression of lipolysis resulting in increased free fatty acid fluxes.

An additional factor affecting insulin sensitivity is the sex hormone profile. The landmark paper by Goran et al. described the transient yet substantial reduction (of ~33%) of whole body insulin sensitivity in midpuberty compared to prepuberty.[25] Of note, midpuberty is associated with a substantial reduction in insulin sensitivity similar to that observed during late pregnancy.[26] The mechanism underlying this phenomenon is probably that midpubertal insulin resistance is aimed at inducing a transient hyperinsulinemic state. The resistance to insulin in midpuberty is restricted to peripheral (skeletal muscle) glucose metabolism and the resultant compensatory hyperinsulinemia (the result of increased insulin secretion during that period[27]) may serve to amplify the anabolic effects of insulin on amino acid metabolism that are crucial during the growth spurt.[28] In obese adolescents, the nadir in insulin sensitivity in midpuberty recovers at the completion of pubertal

development. Some argue that in the obese midpubertal adolescents, the reduction in insulin sensitivity does not completely resolve.[29] Thus, puberty represents an additional metabolic burden in adolescents who were obese and insulin resistant to some degree in prepuberty and sets the stage for the emergence of metabolic derangements such as T2DM and worsening of cardiovascular risk factors.[30] On the other hand, many obese adolescents manifest prediabetes and an altered lipid profile in midpuberty that may partially or completely resolve once pubertal development is completed.[31] One can argue that if altered glucose metabolism is evident in midpuberty, even if completely resolved at completion of pubertal development. This is a strong indication that the threshold of insulin resistance in which the obese adolescent cannot appropriately compensate by increasing insulin secretion has been reached. Thus future similar reductions in insulin sensitivity (such as pregnancy, acute illness, corticosteroid treatment, etc.) may manifest as hyperglycemia.

It is well established that obese children with impaired glucose tolerance manifest marked peripheral insulin resistance compared to those with normal glucose metabolism highlighting the crucial role of this factor in the development of diabetes.[32] These children also manifest the typical adverse pattern of lipid partitioning described above.[33] This along with normal pubertal hormonal changes and potential exogenous factors that may reduce insulin sensitivity may result in altered glucose metabolism and unraveling defects in insulin secretion.

PATHOPHYSIOLOGY OF β-CELL FAILURE

As indicated above, the majority of obese children are insulin resistant to some extent yet only a fraction of them develop altered glucose metabolism. The β-cells of these children fail to compensate appropriately. Upon facing peripheral insulin resistance, there are two basic mechanisms that allow compensation: secreting more insulin or reducing its clearance from the circulation. It has been shown that lower insulin sensitivity in children with normal and impaired glucose tolerance is associated with reduced insulin clearance reaching a trough that probably cannot be further reduced.[34] At this point, increasing insulin secretion is the only other compensatory mechanism. As glucose tolerance represents a continuum, rising glucose levels, even within the "normal" range, are already associated with subtle defects in insulin secretion, independent of insulin resistance.[35] It has been shown that obese children with impaired glucose tolerance already manifest significant defects in first-phase insulin secretion while second-phase secretion is preserved (in obese children with T2DM, major defects of both phases of insulin secretion are evident).[36,37] Impaired fasting glucose (IFG), an additional prediabetic state, in obese adolescents is linked primarily to alterations in glucose sensitivity of first-phase insulin secretion and slightly reduced liver insulin sensitivity.[33] In contrast, obese children with impaired glucose tolerance (IGT) are affected by a more severe degree of peripheral insulin resistance and reduction in first-phase secretion. Those suffering from both IFG/IGT manifest profound insulin resistance and a defect in second-phase insulin secretion making this combination very reminiscent of overt T2DM. An additional factor that may have an adverse effect on β-cell function is the prolonged exposure to lipotoxicity because of increased circulations of FFAs. This phenomenon may differ significantly between obese children of different ethnic backgrounds (being more prominent in Caucasians).[38]

Once the β-cell faces significant insulin resistance, its ability to compensate will determine whether the individual will remain normoglycemic-hyperinsulinemic or develop deteriorating glucose tolerance. The ability of the β-cell to provide enhanced insulin secretion is determined by its disposition index (DI). This term is the product of insulin sensitivity and secretion and provides an estimate of the ability of the β-cell to increase secretion in the context of specific levels of whole body insulin sensitivity. The relation of insulin sensitivity and secretion is such that their product is a hyperbolic function.[39] Thus, when insulin sensitivity is reduced (due to weight gain, pubertal changes, pregnancy, etc.), the ability of the β-cell to respond is determined by its disposition index. The DI is mostly genetically determined and is probably influenced by intrauterine factors.[40,41] Exposure to gestational diabetes in utero results in a lower DI in equally obese adolescents differing by their exposure, reflecting both the genetic and prenatal effects of hyperglycemia on β-cell programming.[42]

As insulin sensitivity declines, the β-cell needs a stimulus to secrete insulin and respond with an adequate compensation. The β-cell does not sense the sensitivity of the body to insulin directly and needs a signal to convey this information. The most obvious candidate for this role is plasma glucose. Indeed, as the obese adolescents shifts to the left along the DI curve (reduces insulin sensitivity), the burden on the β-cell increases and the allostatic response to maintain glucose homeostasis is a small increase in glucose levels (signaling the β-cell to increase secretion). This increase is evident in both fasting and postprandial glucose concentrations that manifest slight yet important increases.[43] Importantly, these slight increases in glucose appear much earlier than the development of prediabetes or overt diabetes and are evident in obese normal glucose tolerant adolescents.[44] Fig. 1.1 shows the dynamics of the disposition index throughout changes in insulin sensitivity.

ADDITIONAL FACTORS IN THE PATHOPHYSIOLOGY OF T2DM

The "yin and the yang" of glucose metabolism involves insulin and glucagon.[45] Glucagon is secreted from α-cells that are adjacent to β-cells within the islet. Multiple signals affect glucagon secretion including the sympathetic arm of the autonomic nervous system, paracrine effects of β-cells (changes in membrane potential, signals transported via gap junctions), and probably direct effect of glucose levels (definitely in rodents). In postprandial conditions, glucose increases along with insulin and glucagon secretion should be suppressed. It has been shown that obese children with insulin resistance, even prior to the development of prediabetes, have lower suppression of glucagon levels in the face of hyperinsulinemia and hyperglycemia.[17] This defect may manifest "resistance" of α-cells to the systemic/local effects of hyperglycemia and hyperinsulinemia. It is worsened in those obese adolescents with IGT. Of note, the slightly increased glucagon concentrations are already evident in fasting obese children with IGT. Thus, dysfunctional α-cells may be part of the factors involved in the development of altered glucose metabolism in obese children yet further investigations are warranted to determine whether this is a primary defect or a result of β-cell dysfunction.

Gut-derived hormones have a significant role in the modulation of insulin secretion in vivo. The incretins, glucagon-like peptide 1 (GLP-1) and gastric inhibitory peptide (GIP), serve as enhancers of insulin secretion upon exposure of the intestinal lumen to food contents. There is conflicting data regarding the levels and response of incretins in obese compared to nonobese adults. It has been shown that obese adolescents with prediabetes/diabetes have a lower response to GLP-1 levels during oral glucose tolerance tests in comparison to obese adolescents with normal glucose tolerance. This manifests as a ~35% reduced incretin effect compared to obese adolescents with NGT in the face of similar changes in GLP-1 and GIP.[46] Thus, β-cell glucose sensitivity deteriorates progressively in obese youth across the spectrum of glucose tolerance in association with an impaired incretin effect without a measurable

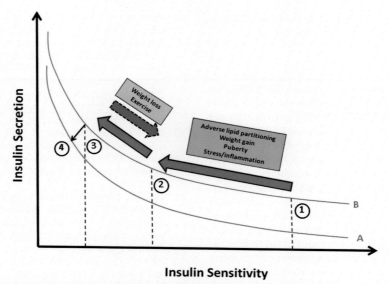

FIG. 1.1 **The Disposition Index, Its Modifiers, and Dynamics.** A (red) and B (blue) represent two different individuals who have a different DI (probably mostly genetically determined). Point 1: Both have similarly high insulin sensitivity yet still, patient A has greater ability to secrete insulin per given degree of insulin sensitivity. Exposure to factors that reduce insulin sensitivity (weight gain, puberty, etc.) shifts both to the left by reducing their insulin sensitivity to point 2. Similarly, patient B can secrete more insulin in the face of this reduced insulin sensitivity. Further exposure to such factors may move both further to the left (point 3). If patient B can adequately compensate by increasing insulin secretion, glucose tolerance will be maintained. If not, patient B will shift down to a new DI curve, closer to that of patient A[4] manifesting β-cell dysfunction. Importantly, increasing insulin sensitivity by weight loss or exercise allows movement on the DI curve to the right for both patients.

reduction in GLP-1 or GIP concentrations. Similarly, other gut-derived hormones such as ghrelin and PYY3-36 have been shown to have receptors on β-cells and to affect insulin secretion[47] yet their role in the development of altered glucose metabolism in obese children is yet to be determined.[48]

Glucose effectiveness describes the mass effects of glucose itself to enhance its own clearance in the context of basal insulin concentrations.[7] Glucose effectiveness is manifested by suppression of hepatic glucose production and enhancement of peripheral muscle glucose uptake and is responsible for more than 50% of glucose disposal in fasting conditions and slightly less in postprandial conditions. As this is an alternative pathway to the classic insulin-dependent glucose disposal pathway, it theoretically could be an ideal compensatory mechanism in cases of obesity-driven insulin resistance. Unfortunately, this is not the case and increasing degrees of obesity over time are associated with reduced glucose effectiveness in obese children.[18] This relation is tightly linked to abdominal obesity.

THE NATURAL HISTORY OF ALTERED GLUCOSE METABOLISM IN CHILDHOOD

In obese children, the trough of whole body insulin sensitivity and thus the most vulnerable period for the development of prediabetes and overt diabetes in midpuberty. T2DM is diagnosed in obese children in this typical age. The natural history of prediabetes in this age group without significant weight loss is not clear. Early studies in obese children with IGT demonstrated that roughly a third progressed to develop T2DM during a follow-up period of ~2 years while a third reverted to normal glucose metabolism while the rest remained with IGT.[49] Importantly, most of those of progressed to diabetes had a substantial additional weight gain during the follow-up. Other studies have shown that a greater proportion of obese adolescents manifesting with IGT in midpuberty will actually normalize their glucose tolerance during conservative follow-up.[50] Importantly, as indicated previously, glucose tolerance represents a continuum. Those with higher glucose levels within the IGT range are more prone to develop overt T2DM over time while those in the lower IGT glucose range are more likely to revert to normal.

CONCLUSION

The metabolic phenotype of the obese child in regards to glucose metabolism is tightly linked to lipid partitioning patterns rather than to the degree of obesity per se. Those with an adverse lipid deposition pattern are more insulin resistant and should be able to maintain enhanced insulin secretion to maintain normal glucose tolerance. Those who develop prediabetes, whether impaired fasting glucose and/or impaired glucose tolerance, may normalize their glucose metabolism in cases where insulin sensitivity improves (such as pubertal maturation) or may progress to overt diabetes if pancreatic compensation fails. It is thus crucial to identify those at greatest risk for the development of diabetes among the large numbers of obese youth and attempt to prevent the deterioration of glucose metabolism as early as possible.

REFERENCES

1. Pinhas-Hamiel O, Dolan LM, Daniels SR, Standiford D, Khoury PR, Zeitler P. Increased incidence of non-insulin-dependent diabetes mellitus among adolescents. *J Pediatr.* 1996;128(5 Pt 1):608–615. PubMed PMID: 8627431.
2. Pinhas-Hamiel O, Zeitler P. The global spread of type 2 diabetes mellitus in children and adolescents. *J Pediatr.* 2005;146(5):693–700. https://doi.org/10.1016/j.jpeds.2004.12.042. PubMed PMID: 15870677.
3. DeFronzo RA, Ferrannini E, Groop L, et al. Type 2 diabetes mellitus. *Nat Rev Dis Prim.* 2015:15019. https://doi.org/10.1038/nrdp.2015.19.
4. Tuomi T, Santoro N, Caprio S, Cai M, Weng J, Groop L. The many faces of diabetes: a disease with increasing heterogeneity. *Lancet.* 2014;383(9922):1084–1094. https://doi.org/10.1016/S0140-6736(13)62219-9. [Epub 2013/12/03]. PubMed PMID: 24315621.
5. Petersen MC, Vatner DF, Shulman GI. Regulation of hepatic glucose metabolism in health and disease. *Nat Rev Endocrinol.* 2017;13(10):572–587. https://doi.org/10.1038/nrendo.2017.80. [Epub 2017/07/21]. PubMed PMID: 28731034.
6. Sharabi K, Tavares CD, Rines AK, Puigserver P. Molecular pathophysiology of hepatic glucose production. *Mol Aspects Med.* 2015;46:21–33. https://doi.org/10.1016/j.mam.2015.09.003. [Epub 2015/11/05]. PubMed PMID: 26549348; PubMed Central PMCID: PMCPMC4674831.
7. Best JD, Kahn SE, Ader M, Watanabe RM, Ni TC, Bergman RN. Role of glucose effectiveness in the determination of glucose tolerance. *Diabetes Care.* 1996;19(9):1018–1030. PubMed PMID: 8875104.
8. Shulman GI. Cellular mechanisms of insulin resistance. *J Clin Invest.* 2000;106(2):171–176. https://doi.org/10.1172/JCI10583. PubMed PMID: 10903330; PubMed Central PMCID: PMCPMC314317.
9. Samuel VT, Petersen KF, Shulman GI. Lipid-induced insulin resistance: unravelling the mechanism. *Lancet.* 2010;375(9733):2267–2277. https://doi.org/10.1016/S0140-6736(10)60408-4. PubMed PMID: 20609972; PubMed Central PMCID: PMCPMC2995547.
10. Goran MI, Ball GD, Cruz ML. Obesity and risk of type 2 diabetes and cardiovascular disease in children and adolescents. *J Clin Endocrinol Metab.* 2003;88(4):1417–1427. https://doi.org/10.1210/jc.2002-021442. PubMed PMID: 12679416.
11. Weiss R, Taksali SE, Dufour S, et al. The "obese insulin-sensitive" adolescent: importance of adiponectin and lipid partitioning. *J Clin Endocrinol Metab.* 2005;90(6):3731–3737. https://doi.org/10.1210/jc.2004-2305. PubMed PMID: 15797955.
12. Weiss R. Fat distribution and storage: how much, where, and how? *Eur J Endocrinol.* 2007;157(suppl 1):S39–S45. https://doi.org/10.1530/EJE-07-0125. PubMed PMID: 17785696.
13. Jensen MD. Role of body fat distribution and the metabolic complications of obesity. *J Clin Endocrinol Metab.* 2008;93(11 suppl 1):S57–S63. https://doi.org/10.1210/jc.2008-1585. PubMed PMID: 18987271; PubMed Central PMCID: PMCPMC2585758.
14. Taksali SE, Caprio S, Dziura J, et al. High visceral and low abdominal subcutaneous fat stores in the obese adolescent: a determinant of an adverse metabolic phenotype. *Diabetes.* 2008;57(2):367–371. https://doi.org/10.2337/db07-0932. PubMed PMID: 17977954.
15. Lettner A, Roden M. Ectopic fat and insulin resistance. *Curr Diab Rep.* 2008;8(3):185–191. PubMed PMID: 18625114.
16. Guglielmi V, Sbraccia P. Type 2 diabetes: does pancreatic fat really matter? *Diabetes Metab Res Rev.* 2017. https://doi.org/10.1002/dmrr. 2955. [Epub 2017/10/05]. PubMed PMID: 28984071.
17. Weiss R, D'Adamo E, Santoro N, Hershkop K, Caprio S. Basal alpha-cell up-regulation in obese insulin-resistant adolescents. *J Clin Endocrinol Metab.* 2011;96(1):91–97. https://doi.org/10.1210/jc.2010-1275. PubMed PMID: 20843946; PubMed Central PMCID: PMCPMC3038472.
18. Weiss R, Magge SN, Santoro N, et al. Glucose effectiveness in obese children: relation to degree of obesity and dysglycemia. *Diabetes Care.* 2015;38(4):689–695. https://doi.org/10.2337/dc14-2183. PubMed PMID: 25633663; PubMed Central PMCID: PMCPMC4370330.
19. Koutsari C, Jensen MD. Thematic review series: patient-oriented research. Free fatty acid metabolism in human obesity. *J Lipid Res.* 2006;47(8):1643–1650. https://doi.org/10.1194/jlr.R600011-JLR200. PubMed PMID: 16685078.

20. Hershkop K, Besor O, Santoro N, Pierpont B, Caprio S, Weiss R. Adipose insulin resistance in obese adolescents across the spectrum of glucose tolerance. *J Clin Endocrinol Metab.* 2016;101(6):2423–2431. https://doi.org/10.1210/jc.2016-1376. [Epub 2016/04/07]. PubMed PMID: 27054297; PubMed Central PMCID: PMCPMC4891802.

21. Roden M, Price TB, Perseghin G, et al. Mechanism of free fatty acid-induced insulin resistance in humans. *J Clin Invest.* 1996;97(12):2859–2865. https://doi.org/10.1172/JCI118742. PubMed PMID: 8675698; PubMed Central PMCID: PMCPMC507380.

22. Yudkin JS. Inflammation, obesity, and the metabolic syndrome. *Horm Metab Res.* 2007;39(10):707–709. https://doi.org/10.1055/s-2007-985898. PubMed PMID: 17952830.

23. Kursawe R, Dixit VD, Scherer PE, et al. A role of the Inflammasome in the low storage capacity of the abdominal subcutaneous adipose tissue in obese adolescents. *Diabetes.* 2015. https://doi.org/10.2337/db15-1478. PubMed PMID: 26718495.

24. Samuel VT, Shulman GI. Mechanisms for insulin resistance: common threads and missing links. *Cell.* 2012;148(5):852–871.https://doi.org/10.1016/j.cell.2012.02.017. PubMed PMID: 22385956; PubMed Central PMCID: PMCPMC3294420.

25. Goran MI, Gower BA. Longitudinal study on pubertal insulin resistance. *Diabetes.* 2001;50(11):2444–2450. PubMed PMID: 11679420.

26. Kelsey MM, Zeitler PS. Insulin resistance of puberty. *Curr Diab Rep.* 2016;16(7):64. https://doi.org/10.1007/s11892-016-0751-5. PubMed PMID: 27179965.

27. Caprio S, Plewe G, Diamond MP, et al. Increased insulin secretion in puberty: a compensatory response to reductions in insulin sensitivity. *J Pediatr.* 1989;114(6):963–967. PubMed PMID: 2524556.

28. Amiel SA, Caprio S, Sherwin RS, Plewe G, Haymond MW, Tamborlane WV. Insulin resistance of puberty: a defect restricted to peripheral glucose metabolism. *J Clin Endocrinol Metab.* 1991;72(2):277–282. https://doi.org/10.1210/jcem-72-2-277. PubMed PMID: 1991798.

29. Moran A, Jacobs DR, Steinberger J, et al. Changes in insulin resistance and cardiovascular risk during adolescence: establishment of differential risk in males and females. *Circulation.* 2008;117(18):2361–2368. https://doi.org/10.1161/CIRCULATIONAHA.107.704569. [Epub 2008/04/21]. PubMed PMID: 18427135.

30. Jasik CB, Lustig RH. Adolescent obesity and puberty: the "perfect storm". *Ann N Y Acad Sci.* 2008;1135:265–279. https://doi.org/10.1196/annals.1429.009. PubMed PMID: 18574233.

31. Reinehr T. Metabolic syndrome in children and adolescents: a critical approach considering the interaction between pubertal stage and insulin resistance. *Curr Diab Rep.* 2016;16(1):8. https://doi.org/10.1007/s11892-015-0695-1. PubMed PMID: 26747052.

32. Weiss R, Dufour S, Taksali SE, et al. Prediabetes in obese youth: a syndrome of impaired glucose tolerance, severe insulin resistance, and altered myocellular and abdominal fat partitioning. *Lancet.* 2003;362(9388):951–957. https://doi.org/10.1016/S0140-6736(03)14364-4. PubMed PMID: 14511928; PubMed Central PMCID: PMCPMC2995523.

33. Cali' AM, Bonadonna RC, Trombetta M, Weiss R, Caprio S. Metabolic abnormalities underlying the different prediabetic phenotypes in obese adolescents. *J Clin Endocrinol Metab.* 2008;93(5):1767–1773. https://doi.org/10.1210/jc.2007-1722. PubMed PMID: 18303080; PubMed Central PMCID: PMCPMC2729183.

34. Weiss R, Dziura JD, Burgert TS, Taksali SE, Tamborlane WV, Caprio S. Ethnic differences in beta cell adaptation to insulin resistance in obese children and adolescents. *Diabetologia.* 2006;49(3):571–579. https://doi.org/10.1007/s00125-005-0109-z. PubMed PMID: 16456682.

35. Yeckel CW, Taksali SE, Dziura J, et al. The normal glucose tolerance continuum in obese youth: evidence for impairment in beta-cell function independent of insulin resistance. *J Clin Endocrinol Metab.* 2005;90(2):747–754. https://doi.org/10.1210/jc.2004-1258. [Epub 2004/11/02]. PubMed PMID: 15522932.

36. Weiss R, Caprio S, Trombetta M, Taksali SE, Tamborlane WV, Bonadonna R. Beta-cell function across the spectrum of glucose tolerance in obese youth. *Diabetes.* 2005;54(6):1735–1743. PubMed PMID: 15919795.

37. Giannini C, Weiss R, Cali A, et al. Evidence for early defects in insulin sensitivity and secretion before the onset of glucose dysregulation in obese youths: a longitudinal study. *Diabetes.* 2012;61(3):606–614. https://doi.org/10.2337/db11-1111. PubMed PMID: 22315322; PubMed Central PMCID: PMCPMC3282810.

38. Michaliszyn SF, Bonadonna RC, Sjaarda LA, Lee S, Farchoukh L, Arslanian SA. β-Cell lipotoxicity in response to free fatty acid elevation in prepubertal youth: African American versus Caucasian contrast. *Diabetes.* 2013;62(8):2917–2922. https://doi.org/10.2337/db12-1664. [Epub 2013/04/04]. PubMed PMID: 23557704; PubMed Central PMCID: PMCPMC3717834.

39. Kahn SE, Prigeon RL, McCulloch DK, et al. Quantification of the relationship between insulin sensitivity and beta-cell function in human subjects. Evidence for a hyperbolic function. *Diabetes.* 1993;42(11):1663–1672. PubMed PMID: 8405710.

40. Rich SS, Bergman RN. The genetic basis of glucose homeostasis. *Curr Diabetes Rev.* 2005;1(3):221–226. PubMed PMID: 18220598.

41. Martin-Gronert MS, Ozanne SE. Metabolic programming of insulin action and secretion. *Diabetes Obes Metab.* 2012;14(suppl 3):29–39. https://doi.org/10.1111/j.1463-1326.2012.01653.x. PubMed PMID: 22928562.

42. Holder T, Giannini C, Santoro N, et al. A low disposition index in adolescent offspring of mothers with gestational diabetes: a risk marker for the development of impaired glucose tolerance in youth. *Diabetologia*. 2014;57(11):2413–2420. https://doi.org/10.1007/s00125-014-3345-2. PubMed PMID: 25168408.

43. Weiss R, Cali AM, Dziura J, Burgert TS, Tamborlane WV, Caprio S. Degree of obesity and glucose allostasis are major effectors of glucose tolerance dynamics in obese youth. *Diabetes Care*. 2007;30(7):1845–1850. https://doi.org/10.2337/dc07-0325. PubMed PMID: 17475938.

44. Tfayli H, Lee S, Arslanian S. Declining beta-cell function relative to insulin sensitivity with increasing fasting glucose levels in the nondiabetic range in children. *Diabetes Care*. 2010;33(9):2024–2030. https://doi.org/10.2337/dc09-2292. PubMed PMID: 20805276; PubMed Central PMCID: PMCPMC2928357.

45. Gerich JE, Charles MA, Grodsky GM. Regulation of pancreatic insulin and glucagon secretion. *Annu Rev Physiol*. 1976;38:353–388. https://doi.org/10.1146/annurev.ph.38.030176.002033. PubMed PMID: 769657.

46. Michaliszyn SF, Mari A, Lee S, et al. β-cell function, incretin effect, and incretin hormones in obese youth along the span of glucose tolerance from normal to prediabetes to type 2 diabetes. *Diabetes*. 2014;63(11):3846–3855. https://doi.org/10.2337/db13-1951. [Epub 2014/06/19]. PubMed PMID: 24947360; PubMed Central PMCID: PMCPMC4207396.

47. Ramracheya RD, McCulloch LJ, Clark A, et al. PYY-dependent restoration of impaired insulin and glucagon secretion in type 2 diabetes following Roux-En-Y gastric bypass surgery. *Cell Rep*. 2016;15(5):944–950. https://doi.org/10.1016/j.celrep.2016.03.091. [Epub 2016/04/21]. PubMed PMID: 27117413; PubMed Central PMCID: PMCPMC5063952.

48. Price SL, Bloom SR. Protein PYY and its role in metabolism. *Front Horm Res*. 2014;42:147–154. https://doi.org/10.1159/000358343. PubMed PMID: 24732932.

49. Weiss R, Taksali SE, Tamborlane WV, Burgert TS, Savoye M, Caprio S. Predictors of changes in glucose tolerance status in obese youth. *Diabetes Care*. 2005;28(4):902–909. [Epub 2005/03/29]. PubMed PMID: 15793193.

50. Kleber M, deSousa G, Papcke S, Wabitsch M, Reinehr T. Impaired glucose tolerance in obese white children and adolescents: three to five year follow-up in untreated patients. *Exp Clin Endocrinol Diabetes*. 2011;119(3):172–176. https://doi.org/10.1055/s-0030-1263150. [Epub 2010/09/08]. PubMed PMID: 20827664.

CHAPTER 2

Clinical Presentation of Youth Onset Type 2 Diabetes Mellitus

ALLISON S. LAROCHE, MD, MPH • GRACE KIM, MD

INTRODUCTION

As we have seen, the incidence of type 2 diabetes mellitus among children and adolescents is increasing. In most instances, making the diagnosis of type 2 diabetes among youth is straightforward due to associated phenotype of obesity and insulin resistance. However, there is an increasing overlap with clinical presentation of autoimmune type 1 diabetes, which can make type 2 diabetes mellitus a difficult diagnosis even for the most experienced clinician. In this chapter, we will review important features of the clinical presentation of youth with type 2 diabetes mellitus including signs and symptoms, physical examination findings, and associated laboratory findings.

Clinical Presentation

Different from type 1 diabetes mellitus wherein patients generally present to care with symptoms of hyperglycemia and in some cases ketosis, the presentation of type 2 diabetes mellitus can be indolent. About one-third of youth with type 2 diabetes present without symptoms.[1] Asymptomatic patients are generally identified from screening of random or fasting plasma glucose, glycosylated hemoglobin, or identification of glucosuria on urinalysis. The American Academy of Pediatrics recommends diabetes screening for youth who have body mass index greater than the 85th percentile for age who also have evidence of insulin resistance, family history of type 2 diabetes, and who are of certain minority racial backgrounds[2] (see Chapter 4 for more information).

The remaining two-thirds of youth with type 2 diabetes mellitus present with hallmark symptoms of polyuria, polydipsia, polyphagia, and weight loss, which cannot be distinguished from those presenting with type 1 diabetes. Up to one-third of youth with type 2 diabetes have ketonuria at the time of diagnosis.[3] This emphasizes the importance of maintaining an index of

suspicion for type 1 diabetes even if the patient has a classic phenotype of type 2 diabetes. Female youth can also present with infectious symptoms such as vulvovaginitis as the first sign of type 2 diabetes as well.[4]

Diabetic ketoacidosis (DKA), as defined by blood glucose >200 mg/dL, blood bicarbonate level <15 mmol/L, blood pH < 7.3, and ketosis or ketonuria, is also common at the time of diagnosis for youth with new onset type 2 diabetes.[5] Among the SEARCH for Diabetes in Youth participants, the prevalence of diabetic ketoacidosis at the time of diagnosis was 9.7% for youth with type 2 diabetes.[6] Sapru cites that 13% of a cohort of patients with type 2 diabetes aged 9–18 years presented with diabetic ketoacidosis.[7] In other populations with high prevalence of type 2 diabetes, 25% of youth with type 2 diabetes presented with DKA.[8] Thus, the phenotype of type 2 diabetes should not distract one from performing an evaluation for diabetic ketoacidosis.

Hyperglycemic hyperosmolar syndrome (HHS) is defined by profound hyperglycemia, hyperosmolality, severe dehydration, altered mental status, and minimal ketosis (Table 2.1).

Hyperglycemic hyperosmolar syndrome is a rare presentation of diabetes, especially in children; however, its incidence may be increasing.[9] The Pediatric Diabetes Consortium examined a cohort of about 500 youth with type 2 diabetes, and about 2% were in a hyperglycemic, hyperosmolar state at the time of diagnosis.[10] HHS can occur in otherwise healthy children, and it is important to recognize, as it is associated with increased mortality. The mortality associated with HHS has been estimated between 10% and 20%, which is a 10-fold increase in comparison to DKA.[11] The indolent presentation of HHS characterized by hyperglycemia, polyuria, and polydipsia may not bring a patient to medical attention early in the presentation. As the fluid losses in HHS can be double the fluid deficit seen in

Pediatric Type II Diabetes. https://doi.org/10.1016/B978-0-323-55138-0.00002-4.

TABLE 2.1
Diagnostic Criteria of Hyperglycemic Hyperosmolar Syndrome

- Serum glucose concentration >600 mg/dL (33 mmol/L)
- Serum osmolality >330 mOsm/kg
- Absence of significant ketosis and acidosis
- Serum bicarbonate concentration >15 mEq/L
- Urine ketone (acetoacetate) concentration <15 mg/ dL (1.5 mmol/L), negative or trace on urine dipstick

Adapted from Zeitler P, Haqq A, Rosenbloom A, Glaser N, Drugs and Therapeutics Committee of the Lawson Wilkins Pediatric Endocrine Society. Hyperglycemic hyperosmolar syndrome in children: pathophysiological considerations and suggested guidelines for treatment. *J Pediatr* 2011;158(1):9–14, 14.e1-2. https://doi.org/10.1 016/j.jpeds.2010.09.048.

DKA, the primary goal for managing HHS is aggressive fluid resuscitation.[5,9] Mortality from multiorgan failure and electrolyte abnormalities is attributed to a lack of adequate fluid resuscitation.[9,11] Complications from HHS arise from increased thrombosis, rhabdomyolysis, malignant hyperthermia, and cerebral edema.[9] In children, it is more common to have a mixed clinical presentation of HHS and DKA in comparison to adults.[12]

PHYSICAL EXAMINATION

Acanthosis nigricans is a sensitive marker of insulin resistance, and is present among 85%–95% of children with type 2 diabetes.[13,14] Acanthosis nigricans is characterized by hyperpigmentation and hyperkeratosis; it appears as a leathery skin change.[15] Acanthosis nigricans occurs primarily on intertriginous areas of the body including the nape of neck, axillary folds, inguinal region, and flexor surfaces.[13] Acanthosis nigricans, when present in pediatric patients, is benign and pathognomonic for an insulin resistant state. The exact pathogenesis of obesity-related acanthosis nigricans is complex. The most common proposed mechanism is the direct and indirect activation of insulin-like growth factor receptor by hyperinsulinemia, triggering dermal fibroblast and epidermal keratinocyte proliferation.[16] In adults, there have been reported malignant acanthosis nigricans on the buccal mucosa that can be markers of malignancy; however, this phenomenon has not been reported in children.[17,18]

Body mass index is a surrogate marker for adiposity, and obesity is closely linked to type 2 diabetes in children. Up to 85% of affected children with type 2 diabetes are overweight or obese.[3] Based on the work from Liu et al., the prevalence of overweight is higher among youth with type 1 diabetes in comparison to the general population thus adding to diagnostic complexity.[19] Visceral adiposity is correlated closely to insulin secretion and insulin resistance.[20] Increased intramyocellular lipid content (fat stored in droplets in muscle) is associated with 2-h postprandial plasma glucose and is inversely related to glucose disposal (the rate of glucose uptake by peripheral tissues such as muscle).[20,21] Measuring waist-to-hip ratios and/or waist-to-height ratios helps to estimate visceral adiposity.[22,23] These indices are commonly used in the research setting, particularly in the areas of T2D and cardiovascular disease. Due to the poor adherence of providers, additional training, and time needed for accurate measurement, the waist-to-height circumference ratio is not a widely implemented clinical measurement. Body mass index is a surrogate marker of adiposity and is commonly used in the primary care setting as a critical risk factor for T2D.

LABORATORY EVALUATION

Initial laboratory evaluation of youth with type 2 diabetes will reveal hyperglycemia as the hallmark. Hyperglycemia can be defined by fasting blood glucose ≥126 mg/ dL (7 mmol/L), glycosylated hemoglobin ≥6.5% (48 mmol/mL), or a 2-h postprandial glucose ≥200 mg/ dL (11.1 mmol/L).[2] See Chapter 4. As type 2 diabetes is a state of relative insulin deficiency in comparison to type 1 diabetes, there are differences in markers of insulin secretion. Plasma c-peptide and insulin levels can be elevated among youth with type 2 diabetes.[24] Nonetheless, in late onset type 2 diabetes, c-peptide levels can be decreased demonstrating an insulin deficient state.

As reviewed in Chapter 1, type 2 diabetes mellitus is not mediated by an autoimmune process as is the case with type 1 diabetes. Thus, pancreatic autoantibodies glutamic acid decarboxylase (GAD), tyrosine phosphatase (ICA-512 or islet antigen-2), zinc transporter 8 (ZNT8), islet cell autoantibodies, and insulin autoantibodies (IAA) are generally negative in type 2 diabetes. In the SEARCH for Diabetes in Youth cohort, 17% of youth with a clinical diagnosis of type 2 diabetes who presented with diabetic ketoacidosis had GAD65 antibodies.[6] Moreover, in the Treatment Options for Type 2 Diabetes in Adolescents and Youth (TODAY) study, about 10% of patients with a clinical phenotype of type 2 diabetes had positive GAD antibodies.[25] Adults diagnosed with type 2 diabetes who have positive pancreatic autoantibodies are considered to be at higher risk to progression of an insulin requirement.[26,27] Pancreatic

TABLE 2.2
Clinical Characteristics of Type 1, Type 2, and MODY Diabetes Mellitus

Clinical Characteristics	Type 1 DM	Type 2 DM	MODY DM
Age of diagnosis	Preschool adolescents	>10 years	MODY2: youth MODY3: adolescent
Obesity	Less common	Common	Less common
Gender	Male = female	Female > male	Male = female
β-Cell autoantibodies	Positive	Negative	Negative
Insulin/c-peptide	Low	High (later can be low)	Low
Ketoacidosis	Frequent	<33%	Uncommon
Associated disorders	Autoimmune dysfunction (thyroid, adrenal, vitiligo), celiac disease	Acanthosis nigricans, polycystic ovarian syndrome, metabolic syndrome	MODY 5: urogenital malformations MODY 8: exocrine pancreas insufficiency

Adapted from Reinehr T. Type 2 diabetes mellitus in children and adolescents. *World J Diabetes* 2013;4(6):270–281. https://doi.org/10.4239/wjd.v4.i6.270.

autoantibody positivity, especially with GAD antibodies, among those with a clinical phenotype of type 2 diabetes remains an area of debate for diagnostic certainty. Patients with monogenic diabetes, also known as Mature Onset Diabetes in Youth (MODY), also have negative pancreatic autoantibodies.[28] Distinguishing type 2 diabetes from MODY, one must rely on detailed family history and clinical features. (See Chapter 5 for more information) (Table 2.2).

COMORBIDITIES

Given the somewhat insidious nature of the development of type 2 diabetes, it is important to recognize that microvascular and macrovascular complications from hyperglycemia can be present at the time of diagnosis. Youth with type 2 diabetes can present with hypertension, dyslipidemia, nonalcoholic fatty liver disease (NAFLD), and microalbuminuria at the time of diagnosis.[14,30] Additionally, comorbidities of obesity including orthopedic issues, obstructive sleep apnea, polycystic ovarian syndrome, depression, and other mood disorders may need to be addressed as well (see *Complications* section for more information).

Risk Factors for Youth Type 2 Diabetes
Age
According to the SEARCH for Diabetes in Youth study, type 2 diabetes is a rare phenomenon in children less than 10 years.[31] The median age of diagnosis of type 2 diabetes in youth is 13.5 years, which corresponds

with puberty during which adolescents are inherently insulin resistant.[14,32,33] The accelerator hypothesis helps explain why there is an increase in insulin resistance secondary to growth hormone and sex steroids play during puberty.[2] In this insulin resistance state of puberty, there is about one-third less glucose disposal observed in teens at Tanner stage II and higher in comparison to prepubertal youth.[1] As puberty starts later in males than in females, the median age of type 2 diabetes onset is estimated to be 1 year later in boys.[31] There are some populations (e.g., aboriginal) in which type 2 diabetes presents in the prepubertal age, which begs the question of if there is a genetic component that may account for the presentation of type 2 diabetes.[34]

Gender
The TODAY study describes a female predominance (65%) among their cohort of youth with type 2 diabetes.[14] The SEARCH for Diabetes in Youth study group also observes a higher prevalence in females.[35] In adults with type 2 diabetes, this gender imbalance does not persist, and the male-to-female ratio approaches 1:1. There is overlap between type 2 diabetes and polycystic ovarian syndrome (PCOS), which is a state defined by hyperandrogenism and insulin resistance.[2] Adolescents with PCOS can have impaired glucose disposal and decrease in insulin secretion in comparison to a non-hyperandrogenic cohort.[2]

Race and ethnicity
Type 2 diabetes is overrepresented among racial and ethnic minority groups in the United States. In the

United States, the highest incidence of type 2 diabetes is among Native Americans followed by Non-Hispanic blacks and Hispanics; Non-Hispanic whites have the lowest incidence of youth onset type 2 diabetes.[31] In a case series of pediatric hyperglycemic hyperosmolar syndrome, African American males with type 2 diabetes comprised two-thirds of patients with HHS.[12] Keep in mind that type 2 diabetes can present in all ethnic groups, and still accounts for almost 15% of all youth onset diabetes cases among non-Hispanic whites.[31] The landscape of type 2 diabetes is not the same worldwide. For instance, in some Asian countries, there are different phenotypes of type 2 diabetes, of which some occur in nonobese children.[36]

Family history

In comparison to type 1 diabetes, an overwhelming majority of children with type 2 diabetes have a family history of type 2 diabetes.[14] The TODAY study observed that about 85% of participants had a first-degree relative with type 2 diabetes.[14] Greater than 75% of youth with type 2 diabetes cited by D'Adamo and Caprio have a first- or second-degree relative with a diagnosis of type 2 diabetes.[37] As type 2 diabetes is prevalent in the adult population, a family history of type 2 diabetes is a sensitive but not a specific marker for youth with type 2 diabetes.

Early life events

Maternal gestational diabetes serves as a risk factor for the fetus' future development of type 2 diabetes. Independent of genetic predisposition, exposure to diabetic milieu in utero is associated with impaired glucose tolerance and defective insulin secretion in adulthood.[38] In the Pima Indian population, which has a high prevalence of type 2 diabetes, children born to mothers with type 2 diabetes were more likely to develop type 2 diabetes in comparison to those born to mothers without diabetes during pregnancy.[39]

Infants who are born small for gestational age also have an increased risk of type 2 diabetes in comparison to appropriate for gestational age infants. Infants with lower birthweights adjusted for gestational age have higher adult adiposity and may experience a modest effect on adult metabolic profiles.[40] One possible explanation for this phenomenon is fetal growth restriction followed by a period of rapid weight gain during infancy and childhood. Others have described methylation patterns of low birth weight infants that can predispose to insulin resistant states in adulthood.[41]

Breastfeeding serves as a protective measure against type 2 diabetes mellitus later in life. The self-regulation of meal boluses in addition to the varied composition of breast milk seems to provide protection against obesity and subsequently type 2 diabetes in youth.[42]

SUMMARY

Youth with type 2 diabetes can have a varied initial clinical presentation, ranging from asymptomatic to more severe cases of diabetic ketoacidosis or HHS. Hyperglycemia, obesity and signs of insulin resistance, and negative pancreatic autoantibodies are hallmarks of the diagnosis of type 2 diabetes. Nonetheless, those with type 1 diabetes are not immune from the obesity epidemic, and there can be overlap in phenotypes between type 1 and type 2 diabetes further complicating the diagnostic picture. Different from type 2 diabetes, comorbidities such as hypertension and dyslipidemia are commonly present at the time of diagnosis of type 2 diabetes in youth.

Type 2 diabetes rarely presents in children younger than 10 years of age, and there is a female predominance in youth. In the United States, type 2 diabetes is more prevalent among ethnic monitories, but still accounts for more than a 10th of youth onset diabetes among non-Hispanic white patients. Family history of type 2 diabetes is ubiquitous among youth with type 1 diabetes. Early life factors, such as gestational diabetes and being born small for gestational diabetes, increase risk for youth onset type 2 diabetes, whereas breastfeeding appears to be a protective factor.

In conclusion, the clinical presentation of type 2 diabetes in youth overlaps with that of type 1 diabetes mellitus. Nonetheless, distinguishing factors such as the obesity phenotype, insulin resistance, and negative pancreatic autoantibodies will help clinicians to correctly identify type 2 diabetes in the pediatric population.

REFERENCES

1. Reinehr T. Clinical presentation of type 2 diabetes mellitus in children and adolescents. *Int J Obes (Lond)*. 2005;29(suppl 2):S105–S110.
2. Type 2 diabetes in children and adolescents. American Diabetes Association. *Pediatrics*. 2000;105(3 Pt 1): 671–680.
3. American Diabetes Association. (11) children and adolescents. *Diabetes Care*. 2015;38(suppl):S70–S76. https://doi.org/10.2337/dc15-S014.
4. Curran J, Hayward J, Sellers E, Dean H. Severe vulvovaginitis as a presenting problem of type 2 diabetes in adolescent girls: a case series. *Pediatrics*. 2011;127(4):e1081–e1085. https://doi.org/10.1542/peds.2010-2311.

5. Wolfsdorf JI, Allgrove J, Craig ME, et al. ISPAD Clinical Practice Consensus Guidelines 2014. Diabetic ketoacidosis and hyperglycemic hyperosmolar state. *Pediatr Diabetes.* 2014;15(suppl 20):154–179. https://doi.org/10.1111/pedi.12165.

6. Rewers A, Klingensmith G, Davis C, et al. Presence of diabetic ketoacidosis at diagnosis of diabetes mellitus in youth: the search for diabetes in youth study. *Pediatrics.* 2008;121(5):e1258–e1266. https://doi.org/10.1542/peds.2007-1105.

7. Sapru A, Gitelman SE, Bhatia S, Dubin RF, Newman TB, Flori H. Prevalence and characteristics of type 2 diabetes mellitus in 9–18 year-old children with diabetic ketoacidosis. *J Pediatr Endocrinol Metab.* 2005;18(9):865–872.

8. Pinhas-Hamiel O, Dolan LM, Zeitler PS. Diabetic ketoacidosis among obese African-American adolescents with NIDDM. *Diabetes Care.* 1997;20(4):484–486.

9. Zeitler P, Haqq A, Rosenbloom A, Glaser N, Drugs and Therapeutics Committee of the Lawson Wilkins Pediatric Endocrine Society. Hyperglycemic hyperosmolar syndrome in children: pathophysiological considerations and suggested guidelines for treatment. *J Pediatr.* 2011;158(1):9–14. https://doi.org/10.1016/j.jpeds.2010.09.048. 14.e1-2.

10. Klingensmith GJ, Connor CG, Ruedy KJ, et al. Presentation of youth with type 2 diabetes in the pediatric diabetes consortium. *Pediatr Diabetes.* 2016;17(4):266–273. https://doi.org/10.1111/pedi.12281.

11. Pasquel FJ, Umpierrez GE. Hyperosmolar hyperglycemic state: a historic review of the clinical presentation, diagnosis, and treatment. *Diabetes Care.* 2014;37(11):3124–3131. https://doi.org/10.2337/dc14-0984.

12. Rosenbloom AL. Hyperglycemic hyperosmolar state: an emerging pediatric problem. *J Pediatr.* 2010;156(2):180–184. https://doi.org/10.1016/j.jpeds.2009.11.057.

13. Fagot-Campagna A, Pettitt DJ, Engelgau MM, et al. Type 2 diabetes among North American children and adolescents: an epidemiologic review and a public health perspective. *J Pediatr.* 2000;136(5):664–672. doi:S0022347600047545.

14. Copeland KC, Zeitler P, Geffner M, et al. Characteristics of adolescents and youth with recent-onset type 2 diabetes: the TODAY cohort at baseline. *J Clin Endocrinol Metab.* 2011;96(1):159–167. https://doi.org/10.1210/jc.2010-1642.

15. Lauria MW, Saad MJ. Images in clinical medicine. Acanthosis nigricans and insulin resistance. *N Engl J Med.* 2016;374(24):e31. https://doi.org/10.1056/NEJMicm1508730.

16. Higgins SP, Freemark M, Prose NS. Acanthosis nigricans: a practical approach to evaluation and management. *Dermatol Online J.* 2008;14(9):2.

17. Fargnoli MC, Frascione P. Images in clinical medicine. Acanthosis nigricans. *N Engl J Med.* 2005;353(26):2797. https://doi.org/10.1056/NEJMicm050300.

18. Wang L, Long H, Wen H, Liu Z, Ling T. Image gallery: generalized mucosal and cutaneous papillomatosis, a unique sign of malignant acanthosis nigricans. *Br J Dermatol.* 2017;176(5):e99. https://doi.org/10.1111/bjd.15396.

19. Liu LL, Lawrence JM, Davis C, et al. Prevalence of overweight and obesity in youth with diabetes in USA: the SEARCH for diabetes in youth study. *Pediatr Diabetes.* 2010;11(1):4–11. https://doi.org/10.1111/j.1399-5448.2009.00519.x.

20. Caprio S, Hyman LD, Limb C, et al. Central adiposity and its metabolic correlates in obese adolescent girls. *Am J Physiol.* 1995;269(1 Pt 1):E118–E126.

21. Weiss R, Dufour S, Taksali SE, et al. Prediabetes in obese youth: a syndrome of impaired glucose tolerance, severe insulin resistance, and altered myocellular and abdominal fat partitioning. *Lancet.* 2003;362(9388):951–957. https://doi.org/10.1016/S0140-6736(03)14364-4.

22. Mokha JS, Srinivasan SR, Dasmahapatra P, et al. Utility of waist-to-height ratio in assessing the status of central obesity and related cardiometabolic risk profile among normal weight and overweight/obese children: the Bogalusa Heart Study. *BMC Pediatr.* 2010;10. https://doi.org/10.1186/1471-2431-10-73. 73.

23. Moore LM, Fals AM, Jennelle PJ, Green JF, Pepe J, Richard T. Analysis of pediatric waist to hip ratio relationship to metabolic syndrome markers. *J Pediatr Health Care.* 2015;29(4):319–324. https://doi.org/10.1016/j.pedhc.2014.12.003.

24. Arslanian S, El Ghormli L, Bacha F, et al. Adiponectin, insulin sensitivity, beta-cell function, and racial/ethnic disparity in treatment failure rates in TODAY. *Diabetes Care.* 2017;40(1):85–93. https://doi.org/10.2337/dc16-0455.

25. Klingensmith GJ, Pyle L, Arslanian S, et al. The presence of GAD and IA-2 antibodies in youth with a type 2 diabetes phenotype: results from the TODAY study. *Diabetes Care.* 2010;33(9):1970–1975. https://doi.org/10.2337/dc10-0373.

26. Davis TM, Wright AD, Mehta ZM, et al. Islet autoantibodies in clinically diagnosed type 2 diabetes: prevalence and relationship with metabolic control (UKPDS 70). *Diabetologia.* 2005;48(4):695–702. https://doi.org/10.1007/s00125-005-1690-x.

27. Badaru A, Pihoker C. Type 2 diabetes in childhood: clinical characteristics and role of beta-cell autoimmunity. *Curr Diab Rep.* 2012;12(1):75–81. https://doi.org/10.1007/s11892-011-0247-2.

28. Pihoker C, Gilliam LK, Ellard S, et al. Prevalence, characteristics and clinical diagnosis of maturity onset diabetes of the young due to mutations in HNF1A, HNF4A, and glucokinase: results from the SEARCH for diabetes in youth. *J Clin Endocrinol Metab.* 2013;98(10):4055–4062. https://doi.org/10.1210/jc.2013-1279.

29. Reinehr T. Type 2 diabetes mellitus in children and adolescents. *World J Diabetes.* 2013;4(6):270–281. https://doi.org/10.4239/wjd.v4.i6.270.

30. Dabelea D, Stafford JM, Mayer-Davis EJ, et al. Association of type 1 diabetes vs type 2 diabetes diagnosed during childhood and adolescence with complications during teenage years and young adulthood. *JAMA.* 2017;317(8):825–835. https://doi.org/10.1001/jama.2017.0686.

31. Writing Group for the SEARCH for Diabetes in Youth Study Group, Dabelea D, Bell RA, et al. Incidence of diabetes in youth in the United States. *JAMA*. 2007;297(24):2716–2724. https://doi.org/10.1001/jama.297.24.2716.

32. Zeitler P, Fu J, Tandon N, et al. ISPAD Clinical Practice Consensus Guidelines 2014. Type 2 diabetes in the child and adolescent. *Pediatr Diabetes*. 2014;15(suppl 20):26–46. https://doi.org/10.1111/pedi.12179.

33. Arslanian SA, Kalhan SC. Correlations between fatty acid and glucose metabolism. potential explanation of insulin resistance of puberty. *Diabetes*. 1994;43(7):908–914.

34. Mendelson M, Cloutier J, Spence L, Sellers E, Taback S, Dean H. Obesity and type 2 diabetes mellitus in a birth cohort of first nation children born to mothers with pediatric-onset type 2 diabetes. *Pediatr Diabetes*. 2011;12(3 Pt 2):219–228. https://doi.org/10.1111/j.1399-5448.2010.00694.x. [doi].

35. Dabelea D, Mayer-Davis EJ, Saydah S, et al. Prevalence of type 1 and type 2 diabetes among children and adolescents from 2001 to 2009. *JAMA*. 2014;311(17):1778–1786. https://doi.org/10.1001/jama.2014.3201.

36. Urakami T, Kubota S, Nitadori Y, Harada K, Owada M, Kitagawa T. Annual incidence and clinical characteristics of type 2 diabetes in children as detected by urine glucose screening in the Tokyo metropolitan area. *Diabetes Care*. 2005;28(8):1876–1881. https://doi.org/10.2337/diacare.28.8.1876.

37. D'Adamo E, Caprio S. Type 2 diabetes in youth: epidemiology and pathophysiology. *Diabetes Care*. 2011;34(suppl 2):S161–S165. https://doi.org/10.2337/dc11-s212.

38. Sobngwi E, Boudou P, Mauvais-Jarvis F, et al. Effect of a diabetic environment in utero on predisposition to type 2 diabetes. *Lancet*. 2003;361(9372):1861–1865. https://doi.org/10.1016/S0140-6736(03)13505-2.

39. Franks PW, Looker HC, Kobes S, et al. Gestational glucose tolerance and risk of type 2 diabetes in young Pima Indian offspring. *Diabetes*. 2006;55(2):460–465. doi:55/2/460.

40. Wurtz P, Wang Q, Niironen M, et al. Metabolic signatures of birthweight in 18288 adolescents and adults. *Int J Epidemiol*. 2016;45(5):1539–1550. https://doi.org/10.1093/ije/dyw255.

41. Quilter CR, Cooper WN, Cliffe KM, et al. Impact on offspring methylation patterns of maternal gestational diabetes mellitus and intrauterine growth restraint suggest common genes and pathways linked to subsequent type 2 diabetes risk. *FASEB J*. 2014;28(11):4868–4879. https://doi.org/10.1096/fj.14-255240. [doi].

42. Gouveri E, Papanas N, Hatzitolios AI, Maltezos E. Breastfeeding and diabetes. *Curr Diabetes Rev*. 2011;7(2):135–142. doi:BSP/CDR/E-Pub/00061.

CHAPTER 3

Diagnostic Criteria for Prediabetes

GRACE KIM, MD

In 1979, the US National Diabetes Group recommended the category of impaired glucose tolerance (IGT) to signify a state of increased risk of progressing to diabetes, although it was also noted that many patients would revert to normal glucose tolerance.[1] This term was created to remove the stigma associated with the other terms in use at the time, and to denote the range between normal and diabetes.

In 1997 and 2003, the Expert Committee on Diagnosis and Classification of Diabetes Mellitus recognized an intermediate group of individuals who do not meet the criteria for diabetes, but this group has a higher glucose level than those categorized as normal.[2] This group was classified as having impaired fasting glucose.[2] Impaired fasting glucose and impaired glucose tolerance are an intermediate stage in the natural history of diabetes mellitus. Impaired fasting plasma glucose (IFG) is defined as glucose levels of 100–125 mg/ dL in a fasting person. Impaired glucose tolerance (IGT) is defined as 2-h glucose levels of 140-199mg/dL during the oral glucose tolerance test (OGTT).

In 2003, American Diabetes Association (ADA) Expert Committee report reduced the fasting glucose cut point from 110 to 100 mg/dL. This was based on receiver operating characteristic (ROC) curve analyses of Pima Indians, Mauritius, San Antonio, and Hoorn studies. The data identified baseline fasting glucoses that correlated with the highest sensitivity and specificity in predicting diabetes over a 5-year period. ROC curve analysis indicated a cut point of 97–99 mg/dL.[1]

This IFG cut point change was to ensure that the prevalence of IFG was similar to that of IGT.[2] This decision proved controversial because it resulted in a 2–4-fold increase in the prevalence of IFG, creating a "prediabetes pandemic".[3] For example, in the Atherosclerosis Risk in Communities (ARIC) study, a fasting glucose of ≥100g/dL had a sensitivity of 70% in predicting diabetes compared to a sensitivity of 50% for a fasting glucose of ≥106 mg/dL. This increased sensitivity generated an increased number of people being identified as abnormal (40 vs. 20%).

Increasing fasting glucose in the nondiabetic range is associated with increased risk of fatal and nonfatal cardiovascular disease. However, the level at which the risk begins to increase differed between studies. From 12 studies, cardiovascular events increased when the fasting glucose was greater than 99 mg/dL. The Diabetes Epidemiology: Collaborative analysis of Diagnostic criteria in Europe (DECODE) study showed the lowest rate of mortality and fasting glucose levels between 81 and 110 mg/dL. The risk significantly increased when the fasting glucose was greater than 126 mg/dL.[4]

However, the World Health Organization (WHO) did not adopt this change in definition of IFG.[1] WHO reported that there is a lack of evidence of any benefit in terms of reducing adverse outcomes or progression to diabetes and people identified by fasting glucose of 100 mg/dL have a favorable cardiovascular risk profile and only half the risk of developing diabetes compared to those above current WHO cut point. The WHO cut point for IFG is 110–125 mg/dL.

The 2-h plasma glucose cut point of 140–199 mg/dL was derived from Pima Indians, which examined the risk of incident diabetes.[1] The incidence ranged from less than 2.0%/year in those with 2-h plasma glucose of <101 mg/dL to 6.8%/year in those with 2-h plasma glucose of 141–198 mg/dL. Another analysis of six prospective studies showed incidence rates of diabetes with IGT that ranged from 35.8 to 87.3/1000 person-years. The rates increased with higher fasting glucose and body mass index (BMI).[1]

There has been relatively little research on the appropriateness of 2-h plasma glucose of 140 mg/dL for defining IGT. The risk for diabetes in Pima Indians is markedly higher at upper 10% of glycemic distribution. The 5-year incidence rate for diabetes was 24% for IGT compared with 4% in people with 2-h plasma glucose <140 mg/dL. There is no consistent threshold for 2-h plasma glucose and adverse outcomes. Increasing 2-h plasma glucose across diabetes and nondiabetes ranges is associated with increased risk of fatal and nonfatal cardiovascular disease. Cardiovascular events appeared to increase in a linear fashion with postchallenge plasma glucose in the nondiabetes range without a threshold, or in a J-shaped relationship with lowest observed death rates centered on 90 mg/dL for 2-h glucose for all-cause mortality and 108 mg/dL for coronary heart disease death. The DECODE study reported J-shaped relationship between all cause and noncardiovascular mortality and glucose with lowest rates at 2-h plasma glucose of 81–99 mg/dL and a graded

Pediatric Type II Diabetes. https://doi.org/10.1016/B978-0-323-55138-0.00003-6

relationship between cardiovascular disease and 2-h plasma glucose.[4] The DECODE study showed that subjects with a 2-h plasma glucose of 180–199 mg/dL had mortality risk similar to those diabetic subjects defined by a fasting plasma glucose of ≥126 mg/dL. It is important to note that the risk for future diabetes, premature mortality, and cardiovascular disease begins to increase when 2-h plasma glucose is less than the IGT range.[1]

The prevalence of IGT was examined in a multiethnic clinic-based population of 55 obese children and 112 obese adolescents.[5] Regardless of ethnicity, IGT was detected in 25% of obese children and 21% of obese adolescents. Type 2 diabetes (T2D) was found in 4% of obese adolescents. In a previous longitudinal study, 102 obese children and adolescent were monitored from a pediatric weight management clinic; 71 subjects had normal glucose tolerance (NGT) and 31 subjects had IGT with repeating the oral glucose tolerance testing after 18–24 months.[6] Six of the participants with normal glucose tolerance progressed to IGT. Ten participants (32.3%) with IGT developed T2D, 10 (32.3%) converted to normal glucose tolerance, and 11 remained with IGT impaired (36.4%). Transition from NGT to IGT to T2D was associated with significant increase in weight, while conversion from IGT to NGT was associated with the least amount of weight gain. The increased degree of obesity and continuous weight gain will have an independent effect on levels of glycemia, independent of changes in insulin sensitivity or βcell demand. The children who progressed from NGT to IGT had the largest increase in body weight and an increase in relative adiposity. IGT subjects who converted back to NGT had minimal increases in body weight and a reduction in BMI z score.[6]

Hemoglobin A1c (A1c) is used commonly to diagnose diabetes. It is also used to identify people who are at higher risk for developing diabetes in the future.

When recommending the use of A1c to diagnosis diabetes in its 2009 report, the International Expert Committee emphasized the continuum of risk for diabetes with all glycemic measures and did not formally identify an equivalent intermediate category for A1c.[7] A1c does not require a fasting blood sample. Prospective studies in adults that used A1c to predict the progression to diabetes showed a strong association between a1c and subsequent diabetes.[7]

In a systematic review of 16 cohort studies in adults, those with A1c between 5.5% and 6.0% had a substantially increased risk of diabetes with a 5-year risk of developing diabetes between 25% and 50% and a relative risk that is 20 times higher compared to A1c of 5.0%.[7,8] The group did mention that those with A1c levels greater than normal range but less than diagnostic cut point for

diabetes (6.0%–6.4%) are at very high risk of developing diabetes.[7] The incidence of diabetes in this range was more than 10 times than that of people with lower A1c.[7]

The adoption of A1c criteria has been debated.[8–13] In the adult literature, A1c had lower sensitivity for diabetes diagnosis compared with OGTT or a single plasma glucose.[14] A1c 6.0%–6.4% was not successful in identifying a substantial number of patients who have IFG and/or IGT.[15] When compared with fasting glucose alone, the combination of fasting glucose and A1c created the greatest predictive value for 10-year diabetes risk.[14] At 5-year follow-up, A1c identified less cases of prediabetes at baseline, but had similar predictive value for progression into diabetes as fasting glucose.[16]

In pediatric studies conducted to date, A1c identifies fewer adolescents with diabetes/prediabetes compared with glycemic measures.[8,9,16] Similar to the findings in adults, A1c did improve predictive value of glycemic measures alone after 2-year follow-up in adolescents.[8] Nowicka et al. examined a cohort of obese children and adolescents who underwent an OGTT and also collected A1c.[7] The area under the curve ROC for A1c was 0.81.[8] The threshold A1C for identifying T2D was 5.8% with 78% specificity and 68% sensitivity.[8] This study had concluded that the use of A1c alone in children and adolescents may result in missed or delayed identification of prediabetes/T2D given the limited sensitivity. The premise of this study used OGTT as the gold standard. However, this study did not evaluate metabolic characteristics linked to future diabetes risk.

In a different pediatric obesity study, A1c was compared with insulin sensitivity measures. The participants were divided into two groups: prediabetes versus normal A1c groups. Insulin sensitivity and secretion were measured using a hyperinsulinemic-euglycemic clamp and hyperglycemic clamp. This study showed that overweight/obese adolescents fitting the A1c criteria for prediabetes had signs of impaired β-cell function relative to insulin sensitivity. This study supported the use of A1c to identify youth with lower β-cell function for epidemiological and intervention studies of overweight/obese youth and progression to T2D.[17] For now, the combination of A1c and a glycemic measure may be the best to identify youth who have the lowest or highest risk for future diabetes. Further investigation on the role of A1c in diagnosis of prediabetes and diabetes in children and adolescents is essential.

TREATMENT

Lifestyle interventions and pharmacological agents may be effective in preventing or delaying the development of diabetes.[2] Even in the absence of frank weight loss, IGT may be reversible in obese children through lifestyle interventions that are successful in maintaining a stable body weight during a period of active growth.[6] Treatment modalities for children present a unique challenge, as nutrition education, physical activity, and behavior modification must be targeted to the family. Parents or caregivers are major agents of change. The Yale Bright Bodies Weight Management is a family-based intensive lifestyle intervention.[18] In a randomized study, this intervention could achieve a sustained BMI z-score decrease for 2 years. Insulin resistance as measured by homeostasis model assessment of insulin resistance (HOMA) increased in control group and decreased in Bright Bodies group. Thus, a family-based program using nutrition education, behavior modification, and supervised exercise can lower BMI, improve body composition, and increase insulin sensitivity.

Sponsored by the Children's Hospital Association, the clinical practices for prediabetes screening and prevention of progression from prediabetes to T2D were identified by consensus of the Medical Management Committee of the FOCUS on a Fitter Future (FFF) Group. A literature review and survey were performed. FFF group included 28 children's' hospitals across the United States. Focus on a Fitter Future on T2D prevention supports dietary intervention to manage weight in children with prediabetes, specifically a low glycemic index diet implemented by registered dietician.[19] More studies are essential to assess long-term effects of diet on T2D prevention in severely obese children and adolescents. The American Academy of Pediatrics (AAP) recommends 60 min of moderate to vigorous activity daily for all youth. Although there are no specific pediatric recommendations for exercise specifically to prevent diabetes, the Focus on a Fitter Future committee strongly supports an increased level of moderate to vigorous physical activity for children with prediabetes.

In terms of pharmacological intervention, metformin is a biguanide that has been shown to decrease hepatic glucose production and also increases insulin sensitivity in peripheral tissues. Metformin has been shown to improve insulin sensitivity in adolescents with T2D and girls with polycystic ovarian syndrome (PCOS). Metformin is being used off-label in children and adolescents with obesity, prediabetes, and/or insulin resistance.[19] In the Diabetes Prevention Program (DPP) of adults at risk for T2D, metformin at a dose of 850 mg twice daily showed a 31% reduction in risk of progression to T2D (compared to placebo over 2.8 years and a 58% reduction in the lifestyle group).[20] A meta-analysis from five randomized clinical trials on adults on metformin found a 40% decline in progression to T2D among those at risk.[21] In obese adolescents with insulin resistance, a meta-analysis including three short-term randomized trials of metformin found a reduction in BMI and fasting insulin with treatment.[22] Three other small randomized trials in normoglycemic obese children with elevated fasting insulin showed reduction in fasting glucose and insulin.[23–25] However, none of these studies lasted longer than 6 months.

Among children's hospital obesity programs through the FFF group, 50% of programs indicated that they used metformin to treat prediabetes and the doses prescribed ranged from 500 to 2000 mg per day.[19] Eight of the fourteen respondents reported using laboratory triggers for referral to endocrinology such as elevated fasting glucose, abnormal OGTT, or A1c ≥ 5.7%. Reasons to stop metformin included improvement in blood glucose, decrease of BMI of 2 kg/m², and improvement in insulin. In addition to the use of metformin for prediabetes, 11 programs reported prescribing metformin for elevated fasting insulin, or HOMA-IR in the absence of abnormal blood sugar or PCOS.

CONCLUSION

The definition of prediabetes is fasting blood glucose 100–125 mg/dL, 2-h blood glucose 140–199 mg/dL, and A1c 5.7%–6.4%. Prediabetes is an intermediate state. The combination of A1c and a glycemic measure (i.e., fasting blood glucose or 2-h blood glucose) may be the best to identify youth who are at risk for future diabetes. Further investigation on the role of A1c in diagnosis of prediabetes and diabetes in children and adolescents is essential. The fundamental treatment for prediabetes is to achieve a healthy weight through lifestyle changes (i.e., healthy nutrition and exercise); reversing prediabetes at this state is paramount. Metformin therapy is an off-label use of treatment for prediabetes in children.

REFERENCES

1. World Health Organization World Health Organization. *Definition and Diagnosis of Diabetes Mellitus and Intermediate Hyperglycemia: Report of a WHO/IDF Consultation.* Geneva: World Health Organization; 2006:1–50.
2. Diagnosis and classification American diabetes association. *Diabetes Care.* 2014;37(1):581–590.
3. Valdes S, Botas P, Delgado E, et al. Does the new American Diabetes Association definition for impaired glucose improve its ability to predict type 2 diabetes mellitus in Spanish persons? The Asturias study. *Metabol Clin Exp.* 2008;57:399–403.

4. DECODE Study Group, European Diabetes Epidemiology Group. Is the current definition for diabetes relevant to mortality risk from all causes and cardiovascular and noncardiovascular diseases? *Diabetes Care.* 2003;26(3):688–696.
5. Sinha R, Fisch G, Teague B, et al. Prevalence of impaired glucose tolerance among children and adolescents with marked obesity. *N Engl J Med.* 2002;346:802–810.
6. Weiss R, Taksali S, Tamborlane W, et al. Predictors of changes in glucose tolerance status in obese youth. *Diabetes Care.* 2006;29:1130–1139.
7. Edelman D, Olsen MK, Dudley TK, et al. Utility of hemoglobin a1c in predicting diabetes risk. *J Gen Intern Med.* 2004;19:1175–1180.
8. Nowicka P, Santoro N, Liu H, et al. Utility of hemoglobin a1c for diagnosing prediabetes and diabetes in obese children and adolescents. *Diabetes Care.* 2011;34:1306–1311.
9. Fonseca V, Inzucchi S, Ferranini E. Redefining the diagnosis of diabetes using glycated albumin. *Diabetes Care.* 2009;32:1344–1345.
10. Lee JM, Wu EL, Tarini B, et al. Diagnosis of diabetes using hemoglobin A1c: should recommendations in adults be extrapolated to adolescents? *J Pediatr.* 2011;158:947–952.e1–e3.
11. Olson DE, Rhee MK, Herrick K, et al. Screening for diabetes and pre-diabetes with proposed A1c-based diagnostic criteria. *Diabetes Care.* 2010;33:2184–2189.
12. Malkani S, Mordes JP. Implications of using hemoglobin A1c for diagnosing diabetes mellitus. *Am J Med.* 2011;124:395–401.
13. Misra A, Garg S. HbA1c and blood glucose for the diagnosis of diabetes. *Lancet.* 2011;378:104–106.
14. Selvin E, Steffes MW, Gregg E, et al. Performing of A1c for the classification and prediction of diabetes. *Lancet.* 2011;378:104–106.
15. International Expert Committee. International expert committee report on the role of the A1c assay in the diagnosis of diabetes. *Diabetes Care.* 2009;32:1327–1334.
16. Heianza Y, Hara S, Arase Y, et al. HbA1c 5.7-6.4% and impaired fasting plasma glucose for diagnosis of prediabetes and risk of progression in Japan (TOPICS 3): a longitudinal cohort study. *Lancet.* 2011;378:147–155.
17. Sjaarda L, Michaliszyn SF, Lee S, et al. HbA1c diagnostic categories and β-cell function relative to insulin sensitivity in overweight/obese adolescents. *Diabetes Care.* 2012;35:2559–2663.
18. Savoye M, Nowicka P, Shaw M, et al. Long term results of an obesity program in an ethnically diverse pediatric population. *Pediatrics.* 2011;127:401–410.
19. Haemer M, Grow M, Fernandez C, et al. Addressing prediabetes in childhood obesity treatment programs: support from research and current practice. *Child Obes.* 2014;10(4):292–303.
20. Knowler WC, Barrett-Connor E, Fowler SE, et al. Diabetes Prevention Program Research Group. Reduction in the incidence of type 2 diabetes with lifestyle intervention or metformin. *N Engl J Med.* 2002;346:393–403.
21. Salpeter SR, Buckley NS, Kahn JA, et al. Meta-analysis: metformin treatment in persons at risk for diabetes mellitus. *Am J Med.* 2008;121:149–157.
22. Quinn SM, Baur LA, Garnett SP, et al. Treatment of clinical insulin resistance in children: a systematic review. *Obs Rev.* 2010;11:722–730.
23. Freemark M, Bursey D. The effects of metformin on body mass index and glucose tolerance in obese adolescents with fasting hyperinsulinemia and a family history of type 2 diabetes. *Pediatrics.* 2001;107:E55.
24. Kay JP, Alemzadeh R, Langley G, et al. Beneficial effects of metformin in normoglycemic morbidly obese adolescents. *Metabolism.* 2001;50:1457–1461.
25. Yanoski JA, Krakoff J, Salaita CG, et al. Effects of metformin on body weight and body composition in obese insulin-resistant children: a randomized clinical trial. *Diabetes.* 2011;60:477–485.

FURTHER READING

1. Lee JM, Gebremariam A, Wu EL, et al. Evaluation of nonfasting tests to screen for childhood and adolescent dysglycemia. *Diabetes Care.* 2011;34:2597–2602.

CHAPTER 4

Screening and Diagnosis of Type II Diabetes

CAMILLE MICHAUD, MD

TYPE 2 DIABETES SCREENING IN YOUTH: WHO SHOULD BE SCREENED

With a high prevalence of obesity in children and increasing incidence of comorbidities, the need for diabetes screening of the pediatric population has been acknowledged, and frequently implemented, in the primary care office.[1,2,7,9,10] Knowledge of the presence of this condition in youth and increased screening efforts may, in part, contribute to the measurable rise incidence and prevalence of a commonly asymptomatic condition. With the awareness of increasing diabetes diagnoses, diabetes screening in the youth will continue to provide clinical benefit to children and providers, as well as epidemiological guidance to the entire medical community.[3,4,10,26]

Glucose Metabolism in Children and Adolescents Is Not Static, and Therefore Neither Is risk

Effects of genetic, epigenetic, and environmental exposures at various time points lead to layers of individual risk that may not be overtly appreciated.[1,5,11,14] Population-specific data remain valuable for screening of disease. Early guidelines of pediatric diabetes screening have been developed according to population and adult-based data. Ongoing evaluation has honed subgroup recommendations, and will ultimately provide further data to continue to narrow the focus of initial screening, and long-term monitoring guidelines.[1]

Current guidelines listed in Table 4.1 suggest screening for overweight children who are at the highest risk of type 2 diabetes development:[1,3,4,27,28]

Current published guidelines instruct that evaluation should be started at puberty or after age 10, with repeat evaluation every 2–3 years suggested while risk factors persist.[6,8,22]

Official guidelines on frequency of testing children and adolescents with severe obesity (BMI > 99th percentile) are not available. Additional care should be taken to not delay reevaluation in individuals with glucose intolerance on initial screen, or additional risk factor development over time; as these cases likely have a higher risk of diabetes development within the 2–3-year suggested screening guideline.[14,27]

There continues to be a high level of uncertainty of determining an individual's risk of type 2 diabetes development over time due to the complexity of insulin resistance and its effects during childhood and adolescence, in particular. Insight into outcomes of adolescents diagnosed with impaired glucose tolerance supports the notion that there is less certainty of known outcomes throughout the population. Although outcomes vary, the comparative risk of diabetes development with a history of impaired glucose tolerance is considerably greater than those with normal glucose handling.[5,11,14,28] The greatest clinical indication of imminent progression to diabetes in individuals with impaired glucose tolerance appears to be an ongoing increase in BMI.[5,28] These children and adolescents with additional risk factors (Table 4.1) should be monitored closely. Individual counseling and clinical efforts to reduce risk of disease progression remain important in those with early indication of diabetes risk.

TABLE 4.1 Pediatric Diabetes Screening Criteria: Elevated BMI (>85th percentile) and Two of the Following Risk Factors
Diabetes in First Degree Relative
High Risk Ethnicity (in relative risk order): • Native American • African American • Hispanic • Asian
Signs of Insulin Resistance • Acanthosis • Poly Cystic Ovarian Syndrome
Maternal History of Gestational Diabetes
Treatment with antipsychotic medications • Included as risk factor for screening inclusion by some sources

Pediatric Type II Diabetes. https://doi.org/10.1016/B978-0-323-55138-0.00004-8

<table>
<tr><td colspan="3">**TABLE 4.2**
Threshold for Diagnosis of Diabetes</td></tr>
<tr><td colspan="2">**Diabetes Screening Studies**</td><td>**Diagnostic Criteria for Diabetes Diagnosis**</td></tr>
<tr><td>Fasting</td><td>Serum glucose level</td><td>Fasting blood sugar ≥126 mg/dL (>8 h without intake), or</td></tr>
<tr><td>Random</td><td>Serum glucose level</td><td>Random blood sugar ≥200 mg/dL with symptoms of hyperglycemia present, or</td></tr>
<tr><td>Provocative</td><td>Oral glucose tolerance test; baseline and 2-h serum glucose levels</td><td>Provocative blood sugar ≥200 mg/dL at 2 h after 75 g glucose challenge (oral glucose tolerance test), or</td></tr>
<tr><td>Any</td><td>Hemoglobin A1c</td><td>A1c ≥6.5% (verification required on another occasion in the absence of confirmation by other diagnostic criteria)</td></tr>
</table>

DIAGNOSTIC TESTING FOR DIABETES MELLITUS AND CRITERIA FOR DIAGNOSIS

Table 4.2 summarizes the studies that are available for diabetes screening and diagnostic thresholds in which to make a diagnosis with each study. A hemoglobin A1c measurement can be obtained in conjunction with any of these studies, regardless of fasting state.[1,4,6]

The use of each screening study provides merits and pitfalls in risk assessment and diagnosis of diabetes in any population. The use of any of these markers for ruling-in diabetes is effective. The findings of impaired fasting glucose or impaired glucose tolerance are considered to fall into a "prediabetes" range, but show a high range of variability on repeat measurements and in terms of prognosis of ultimate diabetes diagnosis.[15,16,21,27] Despite the variability of results that may be observed on screening studies, persistence of abnormal results suggests persistence of cardiovascular risk; and therefore should be addressed accordingly.[26–28]

Random Glucose Measurement Benefits and Challenges

Random blood sugar measurement may be considered as a first line screen in individuals that are not reliable to return for fasting or provocative studies.[32] The sample can be obtained and processed quickly as point of care tests for immediate feedback for provider and patient, and reduces need for phlebotomy and laboratory support. Interpretation of elevation in random blood sugars can be challenging however. Individuals with one result in the diagnostic range for diabetes who do not have symptoms must undergo reevaluation. A diagnosis of diabetes can be made if two samples or two different studies confirm threshold values, or if one study reaches diagnostic threshold at the time of symptoms of diabetes.[29]

Inclusion of an A1c measurement with random testing could prove beneficial in accurate support of a diabetes diagnosis. Despite drawbacks in the interpretation of random results, individuals with symptoms or otherwise at high risk for a diagnosis of diabetes should not have screening delayed.

Fasting Glucose Measurement Benefits and Challenges

Fasting glucose data provide a consistent, known state of evaluation for data interpretation, and have been found to show a stronger prognostic risk of diabetes development.[31] Individuals with diagnostic fasting blood sugars, >125 mg/dL, may still be asymptomatic from the hyperglycemia.[1,4,26,27] Early identification of diabetes-range blood sugars on fasting studies can lead to early treatment implementation, and increase achievement of early glycemic control. A second visit to complete laboratory monitoring is not always guaranteed due to patient compliance however, and therefore it may result in no data rather than an intake-controlled evaluation. As fasting glucose tolerance may be intact and impaired glucose tolerance may not be identified prior to a glucose load, fasting studies may still miss those with a rising risk or a present diagnosis of diabetes.[32]

Provocative Glucose Testing Benefits and Challenges

Provocative testing: Oral glucose tolerance test (OGTT) is performed with 75 g of anhydrous glucose in solution, although a lowered dose for young children can be used: 1.75 g/kg, up to 75 g. Blood sugar levels should be obtained at baseline, prior to glucose load and at 2 h after glucose intake. These controlled conditions provide a more comprehensive assessment of dynamic glucose handling. The reproducibility of OGTT results however is not guaranteed, specifically in obese, insulin-resistant children. Some studies have shown only a 30% concordance with findings of impaired glucose tolerance on repeat testing. Confirmation of diabetes diagnosis is still required with a second value in the absence of symptoms.[22,23,32]

A1c Measurement Benefits and Challenges

The hemoglobin A1c measurement provides an average glucose level over the preceding 3 months. It is important to note that the standards of A1c use for diagnosis of diabetes were developed using adult data. It therefore is uncertain whether the same thresholds of abnormal and/or diagnostic range applies similarly in the evaluation of pediatric patients.[15,19,20,29] Studies suggest that comparing A1c and OGTT data show conflicting results in diagnosis of diabetes and risk determination.[15,17,18,32] Among those with a normal A1c, 27% were found to have impaired glucose handing on OGTT. Individuals with a diagnostic A1c for diabetes were found on OGTT to have normal glucose tolerance in 12.5% of cases, and prediabetes in 24%. The greatest challenge in using A1c as a screening tool arises in interpretation of values resulting in the elevated risk range, as about half of these individuals were noted on OGTT to have normal glucose tolerance, and the other half had diabetes or impaired glucose tolerance.[15]

Caution must also be used in various circumstances in which the A1c measurement accuracy may be affected. Conditions that commonly under report glycemic control (i.e., result in lower A1c on measurement) include chronic anemias, hemoglobinopathies, and cystic fibrosis. Different assay techniques of A1c determination may be affected to different degrees by these underlying conditions; particularly the hemoglobinopathies. It has also been recognized that there a measurable difference in A1c interpretation of glycemia among different ethnicities. African-American individuals with and without diabetes have higher A1c measurements with the same glycemic control.[15,20,29,30]

Inclusion of insulin and c-peptide levels can be helpful information to include in work-up of diabetes, particularly, to a degree, in efforts to distinguish type 1 and type 2 diabetes mellitus. These measurements are not diagnostic for diabetes as independent markers. Individuals with glucose toxicity in both type 1 diabetes and type 2 diabetes may have low insulin and c-peptide levels. Elevated insulin levels in the setting of hyperglycemia would help to confirm a diagnosis of type 2 diabetes. A measurable c-peptide value during the type 1 diabetes honeymoon period should be interpreted with caution, as endogenous insulin secretion remains present for a period of time.[26] Updated obesity guidelines however indicate that insulin levels specifically should not be included in baseline screening efforts due to the vast range of results noted on screening studies and the common occurrence of insulin resistance during adolescence.[22]

TABLE 4.3
Prediabetes Glucose Criteria

| Fasting Glucose 100–125 mg/dL |
| 2-h Glucose measurement on OGTT of 140–199 mg/dL |

Diagnosis of Prediabetes

The term "prediabetes" has been casually employed in cases of any abnormality noted on laboratory evaluation for diabetes (abnormal glucose, insulin, or A1c measurement) or when acanthosis nigricans is noted on examination. The term of prediabetes is easy to understand for the lay population, and can be used to motivate lifestyle change that may reduce overall risk of diabetes and other obesity-related comorbidities. Because of its widespread use in this context however, it has become a less accurate descriptive term in the medical community.

A more accurate determination of a true prediabetes state would be the presence of fasting glucose intolerance and/or impaired glucose tolerance, as indicated by values in Table 4.3.[1,4,5]

Guidelines consistently note that an A1c measurement less than 5.7% as normal, greater than 6.4% as diagnostic for diabetes, and anywhere in between 5.7% and 6.4% as increase in diabetes risk.

The reference range of A1c measurements however are determined based on adult data, rather than established pediatric-specific norms. Observations have been made regarding varying normal A1c ranges throughout different ages and ethnicities.[16,30] Other studies have reported both under and overreporting of diabetes using A1c and OGTT data comparison, and an overall cost inefficiency with use of A1c for diabetes screening alone.[15]

Intervention with lifestyle counseling at the stage of prediabetes is necessary, but no current guidelines exist on the timing and frequency of repeat monitoring. Experts in the field agree that additional information is essential regarding long-term monitoring of the prediabetes state, while unanimously noting need for lifestyle intervention to reduce features of risk for progression of disease.[4,26,28]

Adult guidelines of annual reevaluation are not appropriate for the pediatric population, as rates of progression to a diagnosis of diabetes over the following year are 10% for adults and about 30% in adolescents.[14,26] With more aggressive progression to a diabetes diagnosis and long-term cardiovascular risks noted in those who remain in prediabetes stage, laboratory monitoring at the same frequency in our prediabetes population as those with a confirmed diabetes diagnosis may prove prudent.[28]

Differentiating the Diagnosis: Type 1, Type 2, Or Something Else? Special Considerations

Once a diagnosis of diabetes mellitus has been established, determination of type of diabetes remains important to dictate treatment course and long-term screening of comorbidities. Although increasing incidence of type 2 diabetes has been observed, the more common diagnosis made in the pediatric population continues at present to be type 1 diabetes. Individuals with risk factors for type 2 diabetes are commonly ultimately diagnosed with type 1 diabetes. The mislabeling of obese adolescents with type 1 diabetes has been variable, with studies showing on average 25% of individuals considered to have a type 2 diabetes diagnosis based on feature of obesity, did have positive type 1 diabetes autoimmune markers on screening. In some reviews however, this misdiagnosis increases to 75%.[4,12,13]

All individuals presenting for acute care of symptomatic hyperglycemia should have type 1 diabetes antibody markers screened. Individuals with a low c-peptide, a less severe BMI elevations, have a history of additional autoimmunity, and who are prepubertal are more commonly confirmed to have type 1 diabetes on antibody screening. Clinical judgment remains important in dictating antibody-screening need in individuals with a presentation consistent with type 2 diabetes, particularly with the incidence of obesity increasing throughout the population.

Diagnostic difficulties do arise in patients with characteristics of both type 1 and type 2 diabetes, such as early type 1 diagnoses with insulin resistance, presence of low level positivity of type 1 diabetes antibody markers in type 2 diabetes, and Monogenic Diabetes of Youth (MODY).[4,25,29]

Glycemic control can improve in early type 1 diabetes in individuals with insulin resistance after initiation of metformin use. Due to risk for type 2 diabetes in the setting of obesity, these individuals with early type 1 diabetes are more commonly screened prior to onset of symptoms, and identified before critical immune-mediated beta cell mass destruction has occurred. Education at this time is critical to review ultimate full insulin replacement need despite mild findings, and common mislabeling of type 2 diabetes, at the time of early diagnosis.[13,24]

Additional careful diagnostic interpretation is essential when type 1 diabetes autoimmune markers are observed in individuals without true autoimmune diabetes. Some studies suggest that up to 10% of individuals with type 2 diabetes may have a mild degree of elevation in one or more type 1 diabetes antibody marker, indicating beta cell dysfunction and failure risk. Although type 2 diabetes management and long-term monitoring is appropriate in this setting, individuals with type 2 diabetes with the antibody presence more often progress to insulin-replacement need. Insulin auto-antibody elevation after treatment with exogenous insulin should not be used as indicator of type 1 diabetes.[13]

Monogenic forms of diabetes, also referred to as MODY, present more of a challenge in those with suspected type 2 diabetes. Hyperglycemia to diabetes range results from single gene mutations, with the majority of cases due to Hepatocyte Nuclear Factor 1a, Hepatocyte Nuclear Factor 4a, or glucokinase alterations. A family history of non insulin-dependent diabetes and absent autoimmune markers are common findings of MODY. Absence of type 1 diabetes markers in obese individuals with a family history of diabetes is generally considered a classic presentation for type 2 diabetes. MODY is diagnosed in 1%–2% of all diabetes cases. This subset of individuals is easier to identify in the lean, insulin-sensitive diabetes population who have negative antibody markers. In individuals with type 2 diabetes phenotypes, the true prevalence of MODY may be underrepresented.[3,4,25] Fifty percent of the US adult population has a diagnosis of diabetes or at-risk for diabetes.[27] Genetic testing therefore in the type 2 diabetes population for cases of MODY is not a resource-effective strategy in the adult population, particularly when sulfonyl urea medications are commonly used in the oral treatment regimen for type 2 diabetes. Consideration of MODY in the pediatric population could be undertaken if multiple generations or multiple first degree relatives have a diabetes diagnosis made before late-adulthood (usually before 5th decade). MODY cases commonly follow a milder course, with less insulin requirement and lower A1c.[25]

The intention of diabetes screening is similar to other health aims: to make the right diagnosis, in the right patient, at the right time, to implement the right treatment, and limit health risk. Faced with the challenge of changing health features in each individual and in the wider population, judicious evaluation and reevaluation become the most important tools to achieve these goals.

REFERENCES

1. Reinehr T. Type 2 diabetes mellitus in children and adolescents. *World J Diabetes*. 2013;4(6):270–281.
2. Ogden CL, Carroll MD, Fryar CD, Flegal KM. Prevalence of Obesity Among Adults and Youth: United States, 2011–2014. *NCHS Data Brief*. (No 219). Hyattsville, MD: National Center for Health Statistics; 2015
3. Dabelea D, Mayer-Davis EJ, S Saydah, et al. Prevalence of Type 1 and Type 2 diabetes among children and adolescents from 2001 to 2009. *JAMA*. 2014;311(17):1778–1786.
4. Rosenbloom A, Arslanian S, Brink S, Conschafter K, Jones K L, Klingensmith G, et al. Type 2 diabetes in children and adolescents. American Diabetes Association. *Diabetes Care*. 2000;23(3):381–389.
5. Weiss R. Impaired glucose tolerance and risk factors for progression to type 2 diabetes in youth. *Pediatr Diabetes*. 2007;8(suppl 9):70–75.
6. American Diabetes Association. Standards of medical care in diabetes—2016. *Diabetes Care*. 2016;39(suppl 1):S1–S106. Available at: http://www.ndei.org/ADA-2013-Guidelines-Criteria-Diabetes-Diagnosis.aspx.html.
7. Springer SC, Silverstein J, Copeland K, et al. In: *Management of Type 2 Diabetes Mellitus in Children and Adolescents Pediatrics*. 131. 2013. Issue 2.
8. Dean Heather. What are the screening recommendations for type 2 diabetes in Canadian Children. *Paediatr Child Health*. 2009;14(2):73–74.
9. Pinhas-Hamiel Orit, Zeitler Philip. In: *The Global Spread of Type 2 Diabetes Mellitus in Children and Adolescents*. 146(5); 2005:693–700.
10. Temneanu OR, Trandafir LM, Purcarea MR. Type 2 diabetes mellitus in children and adolescents: a relatively new clinical problem within pediatric practice. *J Med Life*. 2016;9(3):235–239.
11. Sinha R, Fisch G, Teague B, et al. Prevalence of impaired glucose tolerance among children and adolescents with marked obesity. *N Engl J Med*. 2002;346:802–810.
12. Klingensmith GJ, Pyle L, et al. The Presence of GAD and IA-2 antibodies in youth with a type 2 diabetes phenotype. Results from the TODAY study. *Diabetes Care*. 2010;33(9):1970–1975.
13. Tfayli H, Bacha F, Gung N. Phenotypic type 2 diabetes in obese youth insulin sensitivity and secretion in islet cell antibody–negative versus –positive patients. *Diabetes*. 2009;58(3):738–744. http://diabetes.diabetesjournals.org/content/58/3/738?ijkey=7928087c7f0ffa0dfcb2dddd3d18e7ff5f287106&keytype2=tf_ipsecsha - aff-3 and Silva Arslanian.
14. Weiss R, Caprio S, Trombetta M, Taksali SE, Tamborlane WV, Bonadonna R. β-Cell Function across the spectrum of glucose tolerance in obese youth. *Diabetes*. 2005;54(6):1735–1743.
15. Nowicka P, Santoro N, Liu H, et al. Utility of hemoglobin A1c for diagnosing prediabetes and diabetes in obese children and adolescents. *Diabetes Care*. 2011;34(6):1306–1311.
16. Saaddine JB, Faggot-Campagna A, Rolka D, et al. Distribution of HbA1c levels For children and young adults in the U.S. *Diabetes Care*. 2002;25:1326–1330.
17. Al Amiri E, Abdullatif M, Abdulle A, et al. The prevalence, risk factors, and screening measure for prediabetes and diabetes among Emirati overweight/obese children and adolescents. *BMC Public Health*. 2015;15:1298.
18. Lee JM, Eason A, Nelson C, Kazzi N G, Cowan AE, Tarini BA. Screening practices for identifying type 2 diabetes in adolescents. *J Adolesc Health*. 2014;54(2):139–143.
19. Schwartz KL, Monsur JC, Bartoces MG, West PA, Victoria NA. Correlation of same-visit HbA1c test with laboratory-based measurements: A MetroNet study. *BMC Fam Pract*. 2005;6:28.
20. Lee M, Wu EL, Tarini B, Herman WH. Diagnosis of diabetes using hemoglobin A1c: should recommendations in adults be extrapolated to adolescents? *J Pediatr*. 2011;158(6):947–952.
21. Kester LM, Hilde H, Hannon TS. Using hemoglobin A1c for prediabetes and diabetes diagnosis in adolescents: can adult recommendations be upheld for pediatric use? *J Adolesc Health*. 2012;50(4):321–323.
22. Styne DM, Arslanian SA, Connor EL, et al. Pediatric obesity-assessment, treatment, and prevention: an endocrine society clinical practice guideline. *J Clin Endocrinol Metab*. 2017;102(3):709–757.
23. Libman IM, Barinas-Mitchell E, Bartucci A, Robertson R, Arslanian S. Reproducibility of the oral glucose tolerance test in overweight children. *J Clin Endocrinol Metab*. 2008;93(11):4231–4237.
24. Ahmed FW, Rider R, Glanville M, Narayanan K, Razvi S, Weaver J U. Metformin improves circulating endothelial cells and endothelial progenitor cells in type 1 diabetes: MERIT study. *Cardiovasc Diabetol*. 2016;15:116.
25. Shields BM, McDonald TJ, Ellard S, Campbell MJ, Hyde C, Hattersley AT. The development and validation of a clinical prediction model to determine the probability of MODY in patients with young-onset diabetes. *Diabetologia*. 2012;55(5):1265–1272.
26. Helena W. Rodbard Diabetes screening, diagnosis, and therapy in pediatric patients with type 2 diabetes. *Medscape J Med*. 2008;10(8):184.
27. Garber Alan, et al. Diagnosis and management of prediabetes in the continuum of hyperglycemia –when do the risk of diabetes begin? A consensus statement from the American College of Endocrinology and The American Association of Clinical Endocrinologists. *Endocrinology Practice*. 2008;14(7).
28. Zeitler P, Fu J, Tandon N, et al. Type 2 diabetes in the child and adolescent. ISPAD Clinical Practice Consensus Guidelines 2014 Compendium. *Pediatric Diabetes*. 2014;15(suppl 20):26–46.
29. Classification and diagnosis of diabetes. *Diabetes Care*. 2015;38(suppl 1):S8–S16.
30. Berganstal, et al. Racial differences in the relationship of glucose concentrations and hemoglobin A1c levels. *Ann Intern Med*. 2017;167(2):95–102.
31. Shah S, Kublaoui BM, Oden JD, White PC. Screening for type 2 diabetes in obese youth. *Pediatrics*. 2009;124(2):573–579.
32. Lee J, Gebremariam A, Wu E, LaRose J, Gurney J. Evaluation of nonfasting tests to screen for childhood and adolescent dysglycemia. *Diabetes Care*. December 2011;34.

CHAPTER 5

The Role of Monogenic Diabetes in Pediatric Type 2 Diabetes

SUSAN TUCKER, MD • LOUIS PHILIPSON, MD, PHD • ROCHELLE NAYLOR, MD

BACKGROUND

Monogenic forms of diabetes must be considered in the differential diagnosis of pediatric diabetes, and particularly in the presence of insulin independence, when classification as type 2 diabetes is being questioned. Monogenic diabetes mellitus is a group of disorders in which a single gene mutation is sufficient to cause disease. Affected genes are involved in the formation and stability of normal pancreatic β-cell mass, the insulin secretory capacity of those cells, glucose sensing in the pancreas and liver, and in the hormonal regulation of these processes.[1-3] Monogenic diabetes mutations can be transmitted by multiple inheritance patterns, including autosomal dominant, autosomal recessive, X-linked, uniparental disomy, defective methylation, and mitochrondrial, or can occur de novo. Depending on the affected gene and the causative mutation, a person with monogenic diabetes can manifest symptoms at any time from the immediate neonatal period to adulthood.

Maturity-onset diabetes of the young (MODY) is the most common phenotype of monogenic diabetes in both children and adults.[1,2,4,5] MODY is characterized by diabetes of variable severity that is inherited in an autosomal dominant pattern. Patients classically lack accompanying features of autoimmunity, obesity, or metabolic syndrome. There may be substantial ongoing endogenous insulin production, which can modify or eliminate the need for treatment.[3,6] Clinical overlap between MODY and the more common type 1 and type 2 diabetes presents a diagnostic challenge. Other forms of monogenic diabetes to consider in the differential diagnosis of pediatric type 2 diabetes include syndromic forms of monogenic diabetes as well as relapsed forms of neonatal diabetes (discussed below).

PREVALENCE

Overall, MODY comprises approximately 2% of all diabetes cases, meaning that 1 in every 50 people diagnosed with diabetes actually has monogenic diabetes.[1] Several studies have looked at the prevalence of monogenic diabetes or MODY specifically within the pediatric population. The SEARCH for Diabetes in Youth Study is a national US multicenter, population-based study aimed at understanding diabetes in children. Eight percent or 1 in 12 children within the SEARCH study who lacked evidence of autoimmunity and had endogenous insulin production were found to have monogenic diabetes due to mutations in GCK, HNF1A, or HNF4A.[7] The authors estimated a minimum MODY prevalence of 1.2% in the US pediatric diabetes population. Systematic population screening within the United Kingdom established a monogenic diabetes prevalence, including MODY and neonatal forms, of 2.5% in pediatric patients.[8] Studies in other countries have largely found a similar prevalence.[7,9-13] Pediatric referral centers may have a higher prevalence of monogenic diabetes.[14,15]

WHY THINK ABOUT MONOGENIC DIABETES?

The three common causes of monogenic diabetes in children (due to heterozygous mutations in GCK, HNF1A, and HNF4A) have genetically targeted therapy that differs from type 2 diabetes management. However, unless monogenic diabetes is actively considered in pediatric diabetes classification, children are frequently misdiagnosed. In the SEARCH study, 94% of the children studied were misclassified as having type 2 or type 1 diabetes, and 76% were inappropriately treated.[7,16] In the UK study, it was estimated that 50% of pediatric patients with monogenic diabetes did not have a genetic diagnosis.[8]

Making a targeted genetic diagnosis can be life changing for affected children and their families. Knowing the mechanism of disease associated with the gene mutation allows for personalization of medical therapy, as well as reduction in the risk of common therapeutic complications such as hypoglycemia. In some cases, therapy can be switched from insulin to pills, or even stopped altogether.

Pediatric Type II Diabetes. https://doi.org/10.1016/B978-0-323-55138-0.00005-X

These changes can greatly improve patients' quality of life. Surveillance for the development of diabetes-related complications can similarly be tailored to the genetic type, as complications are common in some types, and in others they are exceedingly rare. In this way, knowing the affected gene has prognostic implications. Additionally, discovery of a causative mutation in a child allows for identification of monogenic diabetes in other family members, including asymptomatic individuals, who can then be monitored for the development of diabetes based on their carrier status and at intervals based on the likelihood for rapid progression of disease.

WHEN TO THINK ABOUT MONOGENIC DIABETES

Clinicians must be alert to the features that would increase the probability of a monogenic etiology of diabetes in children (Table 5.1). As a general rule, monogenic diabetes should be considered for any patient with a linear family history of diabetes, negative pancreatic autoantibodies [glutamic acid decarboxylase (GAD65), islet antigen 2 (IA-2), zinc cotransporter 8 (ZnT8), and insulin autoantibody (IAA) for those not on insulin therapy], evidence of ongoing endogenous insulin production (as assessed by serum or urine c-peptide), associated syndromic features, or who simply does not fit with classic clinical features seen in type 1 or 2 diabetes.[2,3,17] Although obesity has historically been used to differentiate pediatric type 2 diabetes from monogenic diabetes, a recent study of monogenic diabetes in overweight or obese children detected monogenic diabetes in 4.5% of the cohort, suggesting that this single criterion is ineffective in determining which youth should be tested.[18]

Evidence-based clinical prediction tools have been useful in reducing the costs associated with unnecessary genetic testing, and have a positive predictive value (PPV) that may be superior to clinical suspicion alone.[17,19,20] For instance, clinicians can use an online MODY Probability Calculator, published by the Diabetes Research Department at the Centre for Molecular Genetics at The University of Exeter Medical School and Royal Devon and Exeter Hospital, Exeter, UK. (found at: http://www.diabetesgenes.org/content/mody-probability-calculator), to help identify patients who are likely to have MODY. This calculator considers a patient's age at diagnosis, gender, current treatment, need for exogenous insulin within 6 months of diagnosis, body mass index, recent hemoglobin A1c, current age, and parental diabetes status. It returns a PPV of genetic testing for MODY, recommending genetic

TABLE 5.1
Clinical Features that Should Raise Suspicion of Monogenic Diabetes[13]

- Neonatal-onset diabetes, either permanent or transient, identified prior to the age of 6 months, or between the ages of 6 and 12 months with negative antipancreatic autoantibodies (see below).
- Diabetes onset prior to the age of 35 years in a person with negative pancreatic autoantibodies, including those to glutamic acid decarboxylase (GAD65), islet antigen 2 (IA-2), zinc cotransporter 8 (ZnT8), and insulin (IAA; which is reliable if drawn before or within two weeks of initiation of insulin therapy).
- Personal or family history of hyperinsulinemic hypoglycemia as an infant, with or without macrosomia.
- A linear family history of diabetes treated as type 1 or type 2, especially in three or more generations.
- Diabetes in a parent that is treated as type 1, or a mother with a history of gestational diabetes.
- Lack of personal or family history of autoimmune diseases.
- Lack of high-risk HLA haplotypes associated with /low type 1 diabetes genetic risk score.
- Nonketotic, noninsulin-dependent diabetes without obesity.
- Normal or increased insulin sensitivity, without clinical signs of insulin resistance (e.g., acanthosis nigricans, elevated fasting insulin level).
- Low or no insulin requirement >6 months after diagnosis.
- Evidence of ongoing endogenous insulin secretion more than 3 years after diagnosis.
- Personal or family history of renal dysgenesis or renal cysts.
- Asymptomatic, nonprogressive, mild fasting hyperglycemia.

screening at a PPV of 25% or greater, or at a lower cutoff in patients with high clinical suspicion. The calculator has not yet been fully validated, but may be useful in giving clinicians a ballpark estimate of the value of genetic testing for a given patient.

DIAGNOSING MONOGENIC DIABETES

If a patient has clinical features that raise suspicion for monogenic diabetes, genetic testing from a Clinical Laboratory Improvement Amendments (CLIA) certified commercial laboratory should be pursued for a definitive diagnosis to guide management. The cost of MODY panels has decreased over the years, but it is still a significant expense. However, studies have shown that genetic testing is cost effective due to changes in treatment, decreased complication rates, and improved quality of life.[21,22] Preauthorization for insurance coverage of genetic testing is often required, and denial of coverage may occur, necessitating appeal. In some cases, genetic testing can be provided at no cost to patients and their families as part of ongoing research studies aimed at furthering the identification and treatment of patients with monogenic diabetes, such as those underway at The University of Chicago (http://monogenicdiabetes.uchicago.edu) and The University of Exeter (www.diabetesgenes.org). Clinical or research-based testing should be reserved for patients with a high pretest probability of a positive test.

MANAGEMENT OF MONOGENIC DIABETES IN CHILDREN

Knowing the causative mechanisms responsible for monogenic diabetes allows for tailored treatment strategies. Below, we discuss management of some of the more common causes of monogenic diabetes in children.

KNOWN GENETIC CAUSES OF MODY

MODY is a subset of monogenic diabetes that is characterized by diabetes of variable severity, with an autosomal dominant mode of inheritance. Patients tend to lack accompanying features of autoimmunity, obesity, or metabolic syndrome. Disease detection typically occurs prior to age 35 years. There may be substantial ongoing endogenous insulin production, which can modify or eliminate the need for treatment.[3,6] Heterogeneous mutations have been identified in at least 13 causative genes,[1,2] often with predictive implications to the patient's phenotype (see Table 5.2).

COMMON MODY SUBTYPES
GCK-MODY Causes Mild Hyperglycemia that Does Not Require Treatment
Clinical features
Children with GCK-MODY are classically asymptomatic, and often come to medical attention during routine screening or evaluation of unrelated illness. They exhibit mild fasting hyperglycemia from birth (typically between 99 and 140 mg/dL), mildly elevated hemoglobin A1c values (generally in the range of 5.6%–7.8%), glycemic variability in response to mixed meal tests

that is similar to controls, and may have glycosuria. There is age-related and minimal deterioration of glucose tolerance over time, as occurs in people without diabetes.[6,23–25]

Mechanism of disease
GCK-MODY (MODY2, OMIM#125851) is caused by heterozygous mutations in the *GCK* gene, which encodes the enzyme glucokinase. Glucokinase catalyzes the formation of glucose-6-phosphate. This is the rate-limiting step in glucose metabolism. Glucokinase is expressed primarily in the liver and in the pancreatic β-cell. In the liver, it is involved in glycogenesis in response to postprandial elevations in glucose.[26] Impairment of enzymatic activity in the liver contributes to the mild hyperglycemia seen in GCK-MODY.

In the pancreatic islet, glucokinase triggers a cascade of events that facilitates insulin secretion in response to rising serum glucose. In this way, it acts as the glucose sensor in the β-cell. In the presence of the mutated enzyme, glucose-stimulated insulin secretion occurs at a higher serum glucose level when compared to individuals with the wild-type enzyme. Insulin secretion follows an otherwise normal pattern, as does the hormonal response to a postprandial glucose load, including insulin secretion, glucagon, gastric inhibitory polypeptide (GIP), glucagon-like peptide-1 (GLP-1), and dipeptidyl peptidase-4 (DPP-4).[27]

GCK-MODY is one of the more common MODY subtypes, accounting for 30%–60% of all MODY cases, depending on the age of the population studied. It is more common in pediatric MODY populations, compared to adult populations. It affects as many as 1 in 1000 people.[2,28,29]

Clinical management
Patients with GCK-MODY typically require no pharmacologic therapy or dietary restriction. At baseline, their glycemic profiles mimic the recommended goals in medical therapy, and do so without the increased risk of hypoglycemia posed by pharmacologic treatment.[6,30] A large study of 799 patients with GCK-MODY showed that patients receiving treatment had no improvement in glycemic control, and there was no worsening of HbA1c when treatment was discontinued, indicating that treatment is ineffective overall.[31] This is likely explained by intrinsic counter regulation that is triggered at a higher serum glucose level.[32]

Complications
The risk of diabetes-related complications in people with GCK-MODY is low in comparison to other MODY

TABLE 5.2
Known Genetic Causes of MODY with Clinical Phenotypes and Treatment Recommendations (Data From Multiple Sources – See Text)

Affected Gene (and Protein)	Prevalence in MODY	Clinical Phenotype	Treatment
HNF1A (hepatocyte nuclear factor 1α)	30%–60%	• most common type of MODY overall, especially in adult populations • glycosuria and progressive hyperglycemia, starting with postprandial elevations • very rarely associated with hepatocellular adenomas • rare case reports of CHI in infancy and childhood, with relapse as MODY	Low-dose sulfonylureas initially. May require combination therapy and/or insulin as the disease progresses.
GCK (glucokinase)	30%–60%	• most common type of MODY in pediatric populations and in women diagnosed with gestational diabetes • mild, asymptomatic hyperglycemia, +/– glycosuria • minimal deterioration over time • virtually no diabetes complications • may cause CHI in infancy and childhood, and relapse as MODY • homozygous mutations cause PNDM	Outside of pregnancy with an unaffected fetus, treatment of GCK-MODY is generally unnecessary.
HNF4A (hepatocyte nuclear factor 4α)	5%–10%	• similar phenotype to HNF1A, but more severe • also associated with dyslipidemia • may cause CHI in infancy and childhood, and relapse as MODY	Low-dose sulfonylureas initially, with progression to insulin therapy in up to 30% of patients.
HNF1B (hepatocyte nuclear factor 1β)	<5%	• associated with renal cysts and renal malformations (RCAD syndrome), as well as genitourinary malformations in females • may involve pancreatic atrophy, and/or malformations of the liver and biliary tree • associated with insulin resistance • may cause CHI in infancy and childhood, and relapse as MODY	Some will respond to sulfonylureas, but early treatment with insulin is generally required.
INS and *INSR* (insulin and insulin receptor)	Rare, <2% collectively	• usually associated with PNDM • *INS* mutations may present as MODY later in childhood • *INS-R* mutations are inherently resistant to insulin therapy	Insulin. Clinicians may consider SGLT2 inhibitors as combination therapy in INS-R mutations.

Gene	Description	Treatment

K_{ATP} channel mutations (in the SUR1 component encoded by *ABCC8*, or the Kir6.2 component encoded by *KCNJ11*)	• mutations in subunits of the K_{ATP} channel that, depending on the mutation, may be sensitive to treatment with high-dose sulfonylureas
	• variable diabetes phenotypes, with incomplete penetrance
	  • most common causes of PNDM
	  • can cause TNDM, either of which can relapse as diabetes in childhood or adulthood
	  • can present as MODY in adulthood
	  • can also present as CHI, which can relapse as MODY in childhood or adulthood
		Treatment with relatively high doses of sulfonylureas is often successful in both neonatal-onset and relapsed diabetes.

PLAGL1, HYMA1, ZFP57 (zinc finger proteins)	• causes 6q24-related TNDM, which may be severe initially but typically resolves within months • overexpression of paternal alleles due to paternal uniparental disomy, paternal duplication, or maternal methylation defects (which may be caused by mutations in *ZFP57*) • accounts for approximately 70% of TNDM cases • may relapse as MODY, usually around the time of puberty or during pregnancy	Treatment with insulin is required at diagnosis. Relapsed NDM may require low doses of insulin, but alternate treatments exist.

Others:
• *PDX1* (pancreatic duodenal homeobox 1)
• *NEUROD1* (neurogenic differentiation 1)
• *KLF11* (Kruppel-like factor 11)
• *CEL* (carboxyl ester lipase)
• *PAX4* (paired box gene 4)
• *BLK* (B lymphocyte kinase)
	• caused by developmental β-cell dysfunction
	• Notes:
	  • *PDX1* can be associated with pancreatic hypoplasia or agenesis; milder defects can lead to later presentation
	  • *CEL* is associated with exocrine pancreatic dysfunction
		Insulin.

MODY; maturity-onset diabetes of the young, *CHI;* congenital hyperinsulinism, *PNDM;* permanent neonatal diabetes mellitus, *RCAD SYNDROME;* renal cysts and diabetes syndrome, *K_{ATP} channel;* ATP-sensitive inwardly rectifying potassium channel, *TNDM;* temporary neonatal diabetes mellitus.

subtypes, and is rare overall.[1,33] Patients are able to achieve glycemic targets without treatment, and have stable HbA1c values over time. Due to normal insulin secretory patterns, patients with GCK-MODY also have low glycemic variability, which has been shown to reduce the risk of glucose-mediated vascular damage.[34] A large cross-sectional study (Steele et al., 2014) compared complication rates between people with GCK-MODY, controls (family members without *GCK* mutations), and people with type 2 diabetes. Other than an increase in the incidence of background retinopathy, which did not require treatment, there was no significant difference in complication rates between people with GCK-MODY and controls. Compared to people with type 2 diabetes, when matched for duration of diabetes, people with GCK-MODY had a significantly lower rate of micro- and macrovascular complications.[35]

HNF1A-MODY and HNF4A-MODY are Characterized by a Progressive Insulin Secretory Defect Responsive to Low Doses of Sulfonylureas

Clinical features
Patients with HNF1A-MODY or HNF4A-MODY have a similar phenotype, the latter being generally more severe on the clinical spectrum. Affected people may have normal or mild fasting hyperglycemia at presentation, but different from those with GCK-MODY, they will have significant elevations in 2-h postprandial values. There is worsening of hyperglycemia over time due to a progressive defect in insulin secretion.[26]

Individuals with HNF1A-MODY have glycosuria that presents earlier and is more significant than that seen in those with HNF4A-MODY. Lipid profiles in HNF1A-MODY are notable for elevated high-density lipoprotein (HDL) and normal triglyceride (TG) levels, which aid in differentiation from both HNF4A-MODY and type 2 diabetes.[36] Low levels of high-sensitivity C-reactive protein (hs-CRP) in patients with HNF1A-MODY also help to differentiate it from other diabetes types.[37] There have been rare case reports of HNF1A-MODY presenting with congenital hyperinsulinism (CHI) in infancy or childhood, and relapsing later as MODY.[38] Patients with HNF1A-MODY have a low prevalence of obesity and arterial hypertension.[7]

HNF4A-MODY is more frequently associated with CHI and macrosomia at birth, occurring at rates of up to 15% and 50%, respectively.[32] Diabetes presents in late adolescence or early adulthood.[32,39] Lipid profiles of persons with HNF4A-MODY typically show an elevated low-density lipoprotein (LDL) level, low HDL, and may or may not show a low TG level.[40]

Mechanism of disease
Hepatocyte nuclear factor (HNF)-1α (MODY3, OMIM#600496) and hepatocyte nuclear factor 4-α (HNF)-4α (MODY1, OMIM#125850) are from a family of transcription factors that regulate the expression of genes involved in glucose transport and metabolism, glucose-stimulated insulin secretion, the renal glucose threshold, and the formation of lipoproteins. Heterozygous mutations in HNF1A are also known to reduce expression of the sodium-glucose cotransporter (SGLT2) in the kidney, resulting in glycosuria that may to some extent moderate the severity of hyperglycemia.[41] HNF4A is a nuclear receptor transcription factor that functions upstream of and to some extent regulating the expression of HNF1A, but it also regulates genes involved in the development and function of pancreatic α-cells, secretion of pancreatic polypeptide, liver and intestinal fatty acid binding molecules, and cellular retinol binding protein 2.[42,26,43] These additional roles may explain the more severe phenotype and unique dyslipidemia of HNF4A-MODY when compared to HNF1A-MODY.

HNF1A-MODY is the most common form of monogenic diabetes, accounting for up to 60% of MODY cases. HNF4A-MODY is more rare (5%–10% of MODY cases) and more severe with more rapid progression of hyperglycemia. Both disorders lead to progressive hyperglycemia caused by reductions in β-cell mass and/or function.[26]

Clinical management
Both HNF1A-MODY and HNF4A-MODY will respond to monotherapy with low-dose sulfonylureas. Despite a longstanding recommendation to use low-dose sulfonylureas as first-line therapy,[17] up to 40% of children and adolescents are being treated with insulin alone, which carries a higher risk of hypoglycemia and achieves worse glycemic control.[44] It should be noted that the sulfonylurea dose required is much lower (e.g., 1/4 to 1/2 of the lowest strength sulfonylurea tablet of glyburide) than those typically used in managing type 2 diabetes and patients typically respond with robust insulin secretion while retaining normal or increased insulin sensitivity.[25] This exaggerated responsiveness confers a risk of hypoglycemia, so caution is advised.

The problem of treatment-associated hypoglycemia has led researchers to seek alternate therapies. Meglitinides also bind to the SUR1 binding site of the ATP-sensitive potassium (K_{ATP}) channel, but do so with less affinity than sulfonylureas and with a faster rate of dissociation from the binding site. A randomized, double-blind crossover study in 15 adults with HNF1A-MODY found that a meglitinide (nateglinide) results in earlier and lower peak insulin concentrations and better prandial glucose control.[45] This resulted in optimal glycemic control, similar to sulfonylureas, which was achieved with a lower risk of hypoglycemia. A small case series in three adolescent patients with HNF1A-MODY had similar results.[46]

A small, randomized, double-blind crossover trial in 16 patients with HNF1A-MODY also showed promise for the use of GLP-1 receptor agonists (liraglutide) as first-line therapy, with similar improvements in postprandial glucose levels and a significant reduction in the risk of hypoglycemia compared to sulfonylureas (glimepiride).[24] However, as GLP-1 therapy is injectable, patient satisfaction and thus medication adherence must be considered.

Further studies are essential, especially in the pediatric population, but meglitinides or GLP-1 receptor agonists may be viable options as initial monotherapy or augmentive therapy. It should be noted that all of these drugs are used off-label in pediatric patients.

Due to the concern for increased cardiovascular mortality with HNF1A-MODY, statin therapy is recommended before age 40 years, regardless of a favorable lipid profile.[47] As weight control is the key determinant of the long-term success of sulfonylurea monotherapy in HNF1A-MODY, an emphasis on lifestyle modifications is also recommended.[48]

Insulin may be required in up to 30% of patients with HNF4A-MODY,[33] and up to 20% of patients with HNF1A-MODY.[48] For patients who fail maximal monotherapy, especially those with HNF4A-MODY, it is important to escalate treatment promptly due to the risk of diabetes-related complications.

Complications

In general, the incidence of diabetes-related complications in HNF1A- and HNF4A-MODY is linked to the duration of diabetes and degree of glycemic control.[26,49]

Despite the favorable cardiovascular profiles in patients with HNF1A-MODY, the risk of macrovascular complications (including cardiovascular death) was previously suggested to be higher when compared to patients with type 1 diabetes[50] and to family members without diabetes.[47] Similarly, the risk of microvascular complications (including retinopathy and nephropathy) may occur at a higher rate than in other MODY types,[33] and at a rate similar to that seen in types 1 and 2 diabetes.[17,50] More recent data suggest that all of these risks can be modulated by early identification of genotype, initiation of appropriate sulfonylurea therapy, and use of statins.[48] It should be noted that the

increased glycosuria in patients with HNF1A-MODY is not associated with deleterious effects.

Although HNF1A-MODY is generally considered to be less severe than its counterpart (HNF4A-MODY), it is rarely associated with hepatic adenomatosis and hepatocellular adenomas (HCA).[2,51] It has been postulated that HNF1A also functions as a tumor suppressor, and a germline mutation confers an incompletely penetrant predisposition for the development of liver tumors following a genotoxic event that inactivates the second allele.[52,53] It has also been suggested that patients who develop HNF1A-MODY earlier in life may have more severe mutations and thereby increased risks of developing liver tumors.[51] Routine screening with liver ultrasound is a prudent course of action, as is the avoidance of exogenous estrogen, which is associated with an increased risk of HCA.[53]

Patients with HNF4A-MODY typically have an atherogenic lipid profile, notable for elevated LDL and lower HDL levels. Triglyceride levels may be paradoxically low.[36,40] The resultant risks of micro- and macrovascular complications are amplified if glycemic control is poor.

HNF1B-MODY Accounts for up to 5% of MODY Cases and Often Requires Treatment with Insulin[2]

Clinical features

Patients with mutations in *HNF1B* rarely present with diabetes in isolation. More frequently, diabetes is associated with developmental kidney disease. It can occur with cystic kidney disease, as part of a disorder known as renal cysts and diabetes (RCAD) syndrome.[54] Along with neurodevelopmental and psychiatric disorders, diabetes can also occur as part of 17q12 deletion syndrome, which includes deletions in *HNF1B*.[2] Additional associated anomalies with *HNF1B* mutations may include pancreatic hypoplasia, genitourinary tract abnormalities in females, liver dysfunction, dyslipidemia, hyperuricemia with gout, and hypomagnesemia.[54] Birth weight tends to be lower in mutation carriers, due to reduced insulin secretion in utero.[29] Overall, the phenotype is broad and variable within families.[2,40]

Mechanism of disease

HNF1B encodes a transcription factor, HNF-1β, which plays critical roles in the regulation of glucose transport and metabolism, glucose-stimulated insulin secretion, and also in the embryonic development and later function of the pancreas, kidneys, genitourinary tract, liver, and the biliary tree. Penetrance is incomplete, leading to variable phenotypes within families, and mutations also occur de novo.[2,54] HNF1B-MODY (MODY5, OMIM#127920) is characterized by endogenous insulin insufficiency due to reduced β-cell mass and dysfunction of the remaining β-cells, as well as insulin resistance.[54]

Clinical management

In the majority of cases, early treatment with insulin is required for patients with HNF1B-MODY, due to the association with insulin resistance and pancreatic atrophy.[1,26] Rarely, sulfonylureas have been used successfully.[55,56] Depending on the severity of the mutation, diabetes may present later in life. When diabetes occurs following kidney transplant for congenital renal malformations, clinicians should be prompted to screen for HNF1B mutations.[54]

Complications

Due to gene effects in multiple organ systems, patients with HNF1B-MODY may struggle with exocrine pancreas dysfunction, pancreatitis, fluctuating transaminitis, infertility, developmental delays, autism spectrum disorder, or schizophrenia, in addition to the increased risk of renal failure due to congenital malformations of the kidneys and genitourinary tract.[1] According to a large, multicenter retrospective cohort study, patients with HNF1B-MODY have a high prevalence of diabetes-related microvascular complications, including retinopathy and neuropathy, and macrovascular complications.[56]

RARE MONOGENIC SUBTYPES OF ATYPICAL DIABETES IN CHILDHOOD

Rare Causes of MODY

Collectively, these rare causes of MODY account for less than 2% of cases identified. In some types, as few as two affected families have been described.[57] Diabetes is typically caused by developmental β-cell dysfunction, and/or progressive β-cell loss leading to insulin secretory defects. Except where noted, treatment requires administration of exogenous insulin.

Mutations in PDX1 (pancreatic duodenal homeobox 1) cause a spectrum of diabetes phenotypes and may also include pancreatic hypoplasia or agenesis. Characteristically, patients have small pancreatic islets when disease is detected. Homozygous mutations in PDX1 lead to pancreatic agenesis.[58] Patients with heterozygous mutations (MODY4, OMIM#606392) can have mild and slowly progressive insulin secretory defects that present at a later age than other MODY types. PDX1 is a transcription factor that regulates the growth and differentiation of the pancreas, as well as the homeostatic mechanisms involved in maintaining β-cell mass. In the absence of PDX1, β-cell death occurs by apoptosis, autophagy, and programmed necrosis. A 2010 study by Fujimoto et al. revealed that β-cell death was preceded by upregulation of a proapoptotic protein called Nix (Nip3-like protein X). Mice with PDX1 haploinsufficiency who were also deficient in Nix maintained normal β-cell mass and function. The researchers concluded that the two proteins oppose each other, with PDX1 mediating β-cell proliferation, and Nix mediating a significant amount of programmed β-cell death.[59] This finding has promise for future therapeutic options, although studies will be limited by disease rarity and the overall mild and slowly progressive diabetes phenotype.

Although they are known causes of MODY, few families have been reported with the following:

- Heterozygous loss-of-function mutations in NEUROD1 (neurogenic differentiation 1, MODY6, OMIM#606394), which encodes a transcription factor that regulates insulin gene expression by interacting with the insulin promotor.[41]
- Heterozygous point mutations in KLF11 (Kruppel-like factor 11, MODY7, OMIM#610508), which encodes a zinc finger protein transcription factor that plays a role in β-cell function.
- Heterozygous frameshift deletions in the variable number of tandem repeats (VNTR) region of CEL (carboxyl ester lipase, also known as bile salt-dependent lipase; MODY8, OMIM#609812), which encodes a lipolytic enzyme responsible for normal pancreatic function. Affected patients also have some degree of exocrine pancreatic dysfunction.
- Heterozygous mutations in PAX4 (paired box gene 4, MODY9, OMIM#612225), which encodes a transcription factor involved in differentiation of pancreatic cells.
- Heterozygous mutations in the insulin gene (INS, MODY10, OMIM#613370), while typically associated with permanent neonatal diabetes mellitus, can be associated with a more slowly progressive loss of insulin secretory capacity, which can present later in childhood. This disorder is postulated to lead to β-cell loss from endoplasmic reticulum stress, which can present later in childhood.[60]
- Heterozygous mutations in BLK (B lymphocyte kinase), which encodes a tyrosine kinase enzyme that functions upstream of PDX1 in the β-cell, and thereby alters insulin secretion (MODY11, OMIM#613375)

- Mutations in either subunit of the ATP-sensitive potassium (K_{ATP}) channel can lead to a wide spectrum of diabetes phenotypes, including MODY, but are more characteristically associated with neonatal diabetes and congenital hyperinsulinism (CHI). It should be noted that there are reports of CHI relapsing as MODY later in life when caused by heterozygous mutations in SUR1 (encoded by *ABCC8*, MODY12, OMIM#606391), specifically the E1506K mutation, or Kir6.2 (encoded by *KCNJ11*, MODY13, OMIM#616329).

Relapsing Neonatal Diabetes

Neonatal diabetes mellitus (NDM) usually presents prior to 6 months of age, and in nearly all cases by age 12 months. NDM can be permanent (PNDM), but approximately half of the cases will be transient (TNDM). The most common cause of TNDM is an overexpression of paternal alleles of genes (*PLAGL1*, *HYMA1*, and *ZFP57*) found in the region of 6q24. Diabetes due to 6q24 abnormalities tends to present within the first week of life, but resolves by about 12 weeks of age. Up to 60% of TNDM cases will have diabetes relapse by an average age of 14 years.[61–64]

Relapsed 6q24-related TNDM is usually treated with insulin, but there is emerging evidence to suggest that dipeptidyl peptidase-4 (DPP4) inhibitors may be effective. These patients tend to retain β-cell mass and insulin secretory responsiveness through the GLP1 pathway.[61–64] When caused by mutations in the K_{ATP} channel subunits (Kir6.2 and SUR1), the first-line treatment of relapsed TNDM is a high-dose sulfonylurea. This strategy is typically successful in 90% of mutation carriers.[1,65,66] The median sulfonylurea dose required for insulin independence is 0.45 mg/kg/day (usual range 0.40–0.80 mg/kg/day, but anecdotally can go up to 2.5 mg/kg/day). Again, this is in contrast to the typical doses used in type 2 diabetes and those used in HNF1A- or HNF4A-MODY.[1,25,65,67,68]

CONCLUSIONS

Clinicians need to have a high index of suspicion for monogenic diabetes among the differential diagnosis of pediatric type 2 diabetes. MODY will be the most commonly encountered monogenic diabetes type, but syndromic forms and relapsed neonatal diabetes may also present in the older pediatric diabetes population. Clinical prediction tools can help to identify patients with atypical features who may have a monogenic etiology of their diabetes. Arriving at a targeted genetic diagnosis allows clinicians to tailor treatments based on the mechanism of disease, adequately monitor patients to prevent diabetes-related complications, and achieve the ideal in diabetes management by identifying patients prior to the onset of symptoms. Discovery of each gene involved in monogenic diabetes has added to our knowledge of the many factors involved in the development and function of pancreatic β-cells. As this genetic database continues to expand, so will our understanding of disease mechanisms involved in polygenic diabetes types.

REFERENCES

1. Murphy R, Ellard S, Hattersley AT. Clinical implications of a molecular genetic classification of monogenic beta-cell diabetes. *Nat Clin Pract Endocrinol Metab*. 2008;4: 200–213.
2. Timsit J, Saint-Martin C, Dubois-Laforgue D, Bellanné-Chantelot C. Searching for maturity-onset diabetes of the young (MODY): when and what for? *Can J Diabetes*. 2016;40:455–461.
3. Naylor R, Philipson LH. Who should have genetic testing for maturity-onset diabetes of the young? *Clin Endocrinol (Oxf)*. 2011;75:422–426.
4. Bell GI, Polonsky KS. Diabetes mellitus and genetically programmed defects in β-cell function. *Nature*. 2001;414:788–791.
5. Sh Ø. Incretin hormones and maturity onset diabetes of the young–pathophysiological implications and anti-diabetic treatment potential. *Dan Med J [Internet]*. 2015;62. [cited 2017 Jun 11] Available from: http://europepmc.org /abstract/med/26324089.
6. Carmody D, Naylor RN, Bell CD, et al. GCK-MODY in the US National Monogenic Diabetes Registry: frequently misdiagnosed and unnecessarily treated. *Acta Diabetol*. 2016;53:703–708.
7. Shepherd M, Shields B, Hammersley S, et al. Systematic population screening, using biomarkers and genetic testing, identifies 2.5% of the U.K. Pediatric diabetes population with monogenic diabetes. *Diabetes Care*. 2016;39(11):1879–1888.
8. Pihoker C, Gilliam LK, Ellard S, et al. Prevalence, characteristics and clinical diagnosis of maturity onset diabetes of the young due to mutations in HNF1A, HNF4A, and glucokinase: results from the SEARCH for diabetes in youth. *J Clin Endocrinol Metab*. 2013;98:4055–4062.
9. Irgens HU, Molnes J, Johansson BB, et al. Prevalence of monogenic diabetes in the population-based Norwegian childhood diabetes registry. *Diabetologia*. 2013;56: 1512–1519.
10. Fendler W, Borowiec M, Baranowska-Jazwiecka A, et al. Prevalence of monogenic diabetes amongst Polish children after a nationwide genetic screening campaign. *Diabetologia*. 2012;55:2631–2635.
11. Rubio-Cabezas O, Edghill EL, Argente J, Hattersley AT. Testing for monogenic diabetes among children and

adolescents with antibody-negative clinically defined Type 1 diabetes. *Diabetes Med J Br Diabetes Assoc.* 2009;26: 1070–1074.

12. Wheeler BJ, Patterson N, Love DR, et al. Frequency and genetic spectrum of maturity-onset diabetes of the young (MODY) in southern New Zealand. *J Diabetes Metab Disord.* 2013;12:46.

13. Neu A, Feldhahn L, Ehehalt S, Hub R, Ranke MB. DIARY group Baden-Württemberg. Type 2 diabetes mellitus in children and adolescents is still a rare disease in Germany: a population-based assessment of the prevalence of type 2 diabetes and MODY in patients aged 0-20 years. *Pediatr Diabetes.* 2009;10:468–473.

14. Chambers C, Fouts A, Dong F, et al. Characteristics of maturity onset diabetes of the young in a large diabetes center. *Pediatr Diabetes.* 2016;17:360–367.

15. Delvecchio M, Mozzillo E, Salzano G, et al. Monogenic diabetes accounts for 6.3% of cases referred to 15 Italian pediatric diabetes centers during 2007 to 2012. *J Clin Endocrinol Metab.* 2017;102:1826–1834.

16. Hamman RF, Bell RA, Dabelea D, et al. The SEARCH for diabetes in youth study: rationale, findings, and future directions. *Diabetes Care.* 2014;37:3336–3344.

17. Rubio-Cabezas O, Hattersley AT, Njølstad PR, et al. International society for pediatric and adolescent diabetes. ISPAD clinical practice consensus guidelines 2014. The diagnosis and management of monogenic diabetes in children and adolescents *Pediatr Diabetes.* 2014;15(suppl 20): 47–64.

18. Kleinberger JW, Copeland KC, Gandica RG, et al. Monogenic diabetes in overweight and obese youth diagnosed with type 2 diabetes: the TODAY clinical trial. *Genet Med.* 2018;20:583–590.

19. Shields BM, McDonald TJ, Ellard S, Campbell MJ, Hyde C, Hattersley AT. The development and validation of a clinical prediction model to determine the probability of MODY in patients with young-onset diabetes. *Diabetologia.* 2012;55:1265–1272.

20. Patel KA, Oram RA, Flanagan SE, et al. Type 1 Diabetes Genetic Risk Score: a novel tool to discriminate monogenic and type 1 diabetes. *Diabetes.* 2016;65:2094–2099.

21. Greeley SAW, John PM, Winn AN, et al. The cost-effectiveness of personalized genetic medicine: the case of genetic testing in neonatal diabetes. *Diabetes Care.* 2011;34:622–627.

22. Naylor RN, John PM, Winn AN, et al. Cost-effectiveness of MODY genetic testing: translating genomic advances into practical health applications. *Diabetes Care.* 2014;37: 202–209.

23. Froguel P, Zouali H, Vionnet N, et al. Familial hyperglycemia due to mutations in glucokinase – definition of a subtype of diabetes mellitus. *N Engl J Med.* 1993;328:697–702.

24. Østoft SH, Bagger JI, Hansen T, et al. Glucose-lowering effects and low risk of hypoglycemia in patients with maturity-onset diabetes of the young when treated with a GLP-1 receptor agonist: a double-blind, randomized, crossover trial. *Diabetes Care.* 2014;37:1797–1805.

25. Pearson ER, Starkey BJ, Powell RJ, Gribble FM, Clark PM, Hattersley AT. Genetic cause of hyperglycaemia and response to treatment in diabetes. *Lancet.* 2003;362:1275–1281.

26. Fajans SS, Bell GI, Polonsky KS. Molecular mechanisms and clinical pathophysiology of maturity-onset diabetes of the young. *N Engl J Med.* 2001;345:971–980.

27. Østoft SH, Bagger JI, Hansen T, et al. Postprandial incretin and islet hormone responses and dipeptidyl-peptidase 4 enzymatic activity in patients with maturity onset diabetes of the young. *Eur J Endocrinol.* 2015;173:205–215.

28. Chakera AJ, Spyer G, Vincent N, Ellard S, Hattersley AT, Dunne FP. The 0.1% of the population with glucokinase monogenic diabetes can be recognized by clinical characteristics in pregnancy: the Atlantic Diabetes in Pregnancy cohort. *Diabetes Care.* 2014;37:1230–1236.

29. Gardner DS, Tai ES. Clinical features and treatment of maturity onset diabetes of the young (MODY). *Diabetes Metab Syndr Obes Targets Ther.* 2012;5:101–108.

30. Association AD. 6. Glycemic targets. *Diabetes Care.* 2017;40: S48–S56.

31. Stride A, Shields B, Gill-Carey O, et al. Cross-sectional and longitudinal studies suggest pharmacological treatment used in patients with glucokinase mutations does not alter glycaemia. *Diabetologia.* 2014;57:54–56.

32. Amed S, Oram R. Maturity-onset diabetes of the young (MODY): making the right diagnosis to optimize treatment. *Can J Diabetes.* 2016;40:449–454.

33. Velho G, Vaxillaire M, Boccio V, Charpentier G, Froguel P. Diabetes complications in NIDDM kindreds linked to the MODY3 locus on chromosome 12q. *Diabetes Care.* 1996;19:915–919.

34. Hirsch IB, Brownlee M. Should minimal blood glucose variability become the gold standard of glycemic control? *J Diabetes Complicat.* 2005;19:178–181.

35. Steele AM, Shields BM, Wensley KJ, Colclough K, Ellard S, Hattersley AT. Prevalence of vascular complications among patients with glucokinase mutations and prolonged, mild hyperglycemia. *JAMA.* 2014;311:279–286.

36. McDonald TJ, McEneny J, Pearson ER, et al. Lipoprotein composition in HNF1A-MODY: differentiating between HNF1A-MODY and type 2 diabetes. *Clin Chim Acta Int J Clin Chem.* 2012;413:927–932.

37. McDonald TJ, Shields BM, Lawry J, et al. High-sensitivity CRP discriminates HNF1A-MODY from other subtypes of diabetes. *Diabetes Care.* 2011;34:1860–1862.

38. Stanescu DE, Hughes N, Kaplan B, Stanley CA, De León DD. Novel presentations of congenital hyperinsulinism due to mutations in the MODY genes: HNF1A and HNF4A. *J Clin Endocrinol Metab.* 2012;97:E2026–E2030.

39. Pearson ER, Boj SF, Steele AM, et al. Macrosomia and hyperinsulinaemic hypoglycaemia in patients with heterozygous mutations in the HNF4A gene. *PLoS Med.* 2007;4.e118.

40. Pearson ER, Pruhova S, Tack CJ, et al. Molecular genetics and phenotypic characteristics of MODY caused by hepatocyte nuclear factor 4alpha mutations in a large European collection. *Diabetologia.* 2005;48:878–885.

41. Pontoglio M, Prié D, Cheret C, et al. HNF1α controls renal glucose reabsorption in mouse and man. *EMBO Rep.* 2000;1:359–365.

42. Stoffel M, Duncan SA. The maturity-onset diabetes of the young (MODY1) transcription factor HNF4α regulates expression

of genes required for glucose transport and metabolism. *Proc Natl Acad Sci U. S. A.* 1997;94:13209–13214.

43. Ryffel GU. Mutations in the human genes encoding the transcription factors of the hepatocyte nuclear factor (HNF)1 and HNF4 families: functional and pathological consequences. *J Mol Endocrinol.* 2001;27:11–29.

44. Raile K, Schober E, Konrad K, et al. The Dpv initiative the German Bmbf competence network diabetes mellitus. Treatment of young patients with HNF1A mutations (HNF1A–MODY). *Diabetes Med.* 2015;32:526–530.

45. Tuomi T, Honkanen EH, Isomaa B, et al. Improved prandial glucose control with lower risk of hypoglycemia with nateglinide than with glibenclamide in patients with maturity-onset diabetes of the young type 3. *Diabetes Care.* 2006;29(2):189–194.

46. Becker M, Galler A, Raile K. Meglitinide analogues in adolescent patients with HNF1A-MODY (MODY 3). *Pediatrics.* 2014;2012–2537.

47. Steele AM, Shields BM, Shepherd M, Ellard S, Hattersley AT, Pearson ER. Increased all-cause and cardiovascular mortality in monogenic diabetes as a result of mutations in the HNF1A gene. *Diabetes Med J Br Diabetes Assoc.* 2010;27:157–161.

48. Bacon S, Kyithar MP, Rizvi SR, et al. Successful maintenance on sulphonylurea therapy and low diabetes complication rates in a HNF1A-MODY cohort. *Diabetes Med J Br Diabetes Assoc.* 2016;33:976–984.

49. Carroll RW, Murphy R. Monogenic diabetes: a diagnostic algorithm for clinicians. *Genes.* 2013;4:522–535.

50. Isomaa B, Henricsson M, Lehto M, et al. Chronic diabetic complications in patients with MODY3 diabetes. *Diabetologia.* 1998;41:467–473.

51. Jeannot E, Mellottee L, Bioulac-Sage P, et al. Spectrum of HNF1A somatic mutations in hepatocellular adenoma differs from that in patients with MODY3 and suggests genotoxic damage. *Diabetes.* 2010;59:1836–1844.

52. Bioulac-Sage P, Laumonier H, Laurent C, Zucman-Rossi J, Balabaud C. Hepatocellular adenoma: what is new in 2008. *Hepatol Int.* 2008;2:316–321.

53. Nault J, Bioulac–Sage P, Zucman–Rossi J. Hepatocellular benign tumors—from molecular classification to personalized clinical care. *Gastroenterology.* 2013;144:888–902.

54. Clissold RL, Hamilton AJ, Hattersley AT, Ellard S, Bingham C. HNF1B-associated renal and extra-renal disease—an expanding clinical spectrum. *Nat Rev Nephrol.* 2014;11:nrneph.2014.232.

55. Pearson ER, Badman MK, Lockwood CR, et al. Contrasting diabetes phenotypes associated with hepatocyte nuclear factor-1alpha and -1beta mutations. *Diabetes Care.* 2004;27:1102–1107.

56. Dubois-Laforgue D, Cornu E, Saint-Martin C, Coste J, Bellanné-Chantelot C, Timsit J. Diabetes, associated clinical spectrum, long-term prognosis, and genotype/phenotype correlations in 201 adult patients with hepatocyte nuclear factor 1B (HNF1B) molecular defects. *Diabetes Care.* 2017;40:1436–1443.

57. Ræder H, Johansson S, Holm PI, et al. Mutations in the CEL VNTR cause a syndrome of diabetes and pancreatic exocrine dysfunction. *Nat Genet.* 2006;38:54–62.

58. Staffers DA, Ferrer J, Clarke WL, Habener JF. Early-onset type-II diabetes mellitus (MODY4) linked to IPF1. *Nat Genet.* 1997;17:138–139.

59. Fujimoto K, Ford EL, Tran H, et al. Loss of Nix in Pdx1-deficient mice prevents apoptotic and necrotic β cell death and diabetes. *J Clin Invest.* 2010;120:4031–4039.

60. Molven A, Ringdal M, Nordbø AM, et al. Mutations in the insulin gene can cause MODY and autoantibody-negative type 1 diabetes. *Diabetes.* 2008;57:1131–1135.

61. Yorifuji T, Hashimoto Y, Kawakita R, et al. Relapsing 6q24-related transient neonatal diabetes mellitus successfully treated with a dipeptidyl peptidase-4 inhibitor: a case report. *Pediatr Diabetes.* 2014;15:606–610.

62. Temple IK, Gardner RJ, Mackay DJ, Barber JC, Robinson DO, Shield JP. Transient neonatal diabetes: widening the understanding of the etiopathogenesis of diabetes. *Diabetes.* 2000;49:1359–1366.

63. Temple IK, Mackay DJ, Docherty LE. Diabetes mellitus, 6q24-related transient neonatal [Internet]. In: Pagon RA, Adam MP, Ardinger HH, et al., eds. *GeneReviews(®).* Seattle (WA): University of Washington, Seattle; 1993. [cited 2017 Jul 28]. Available from: http://www.ncbi.nlm.nih.go v/books/NBK1534/.

64. Yorifuji T, Matsubara K, Sakakibara A, et al. Abnormalities in chromosome 6q24 as a cause of early-onset, non-obese, non-autoimmune diabetes mellitus without history of neonatal diabetes. *Diabetes Med J Br Diabetes Assoc.* 2015;32:963–967.

65. Pearson ER, Flechtner I, Njølstad PR, et al. Switching from insulin to oral sulfonylureas in patients with diabetes due to Kir6.2 mutations. *N Engl J Med.* 2006;355:467–477.

66. Patch AM, Flanagan SE, Boustred C, Hattersley AT, Ellard S. Mutations in the ABCC8 gene encoding the SUR1 subunit of the KATP channel cause transient neonatal diabetes, permanent neonatal diabetes or permanent diabetes diagnosed outside the neonatal period. *Diabetes Obes Metab.* 2007;9(suppl 2):28–39.

67. Greeley SAW, Tucker SE, Worrell HI, Skowron KB, Bell GI, Philipson LH. Update in neonatal diabetes. *Curr Opin Endocrinol Diabetes Obes.* 2010;17:13–19.

68. Codner E, Flanagan S, Ellard S, García H, Hattersley AT. High-dose glibenclamide can replace insulin therapy despite transitory diarrhea in early-onset diabetes caused by a novel R201L Kir6.2 mutation. *Diabetes Care.* 2005;28:758–759.

CHAPTER 6

Hypertension and Type 2 Diabetes Mellitus in Children and Adolescents

CHARUMATHI BASKARAN, MD • LYNNE L. LEVITSKY, MD

INTRODUCTION

Type 2 diabetes mellitus (T2D), a diagnosis that was uncommon in children a few decades ago, is being increasingly recognized in youth and adolescents and presents the physician with a unique challenge of managing multiple metabolic derangements at a young age. This increase in T2D rates in children parallels the increase in prevalence of obesity seen worldwide. Overall obesity rates in children and young adolescents appear to have plateaued in the last decade[1]; however, severe obesity continues to be on the rise, posing significant future cardiovascular and metabolic risks.[2] In the year 2011–12, T2D was diagnosed in 12.5 cases per 1,00,000 youth between the ages of 10 and 19 years.[3] This represented a relative annual increase in T2D incidence of 4.8% from 2002 to 2012, after adjustment for age, race, and ethnicity.[3] The SEARCH study for diabetes in children and adolescents estimated an overall prevalence of T2D of 0.46 per 1000 children with higher rates in American Indian, African American, and Hispanic youth.[4] Of note, in this study, the T2D prevalence had increased by 30.5% in youth aged 10–19 years from 2001 to 2009.[4] Young onset T2D is associated with greater mortality rates and long-term cardiovascular complications compared with type 1 diabetes (T1D)[5] underscoring the need to better understand the pathophysiology and management of these complications in T2D.

The alarming increase in all classes of obesity in children has led to the increased occurrence of a group of other metabolic derangements including impaired glucose tolerance, hypertension, and dyslipidemia, commonly linked as metabolic syndrome.[6–8] In this chapter, we will review the prevalence, pathology, and management of hypertension and nephropathy in youth with T2D.

HYPERTENSION IN T2D

Primary hypertension is diagnosed frequently in children. The actual prevalence of clinical hypertension in children and adolescents is 3.5%.[9] High blood pressures in children track into adulthood and adults with higher blood pressure in childhood develop early hypertension.[9,10] Different from adults, blood pressures in children are categorized based on the normative data for age, gender, and height and "hypertension" is defined as a systolic or diastolic blood pressure greater than the 95th percentile for age, gender, and height.[11] Although these standards do not account for the weight status of the individual, studies have consistently demonstrated increasing blood pressure values with increasing BMI percentiles.[12]

Difference in Prevalence of Hypertension Between T1D and T2D

In adults, hypertension is more common in patients with T2D compared with T1D (50%–80% vs. 30%) and is often present at the time of diabetes diagnosis.[13] The SEARCH study and the Treatment Options for Youth with T2D (TODAY) study are two large studies in United States that provide a wealth of data on T2D and its comorbidities in adolescents and youth.[14] The SEARCH Study, a multicenter epidemiological study of youth with diabetes, reported that 5.9% and 23.7% of youth with T1D and T2D, respectively, had elevated blood pressure.[15] Data from an Australian cohort examining 1443 children with T1D and 68 adolescents with T2D showed 16% and 36% hypertension prevalence, similar to the findings in SEARCH study.[16] In another cohort of 699 adolescents with T2D of <2 years duration, in the TODAY study, 11.6% had hypertension at baseline and 33.8% had hypertension at 4 years of follow-up.[17] Males had 87% higher risk of developing hypertension in this study. Furthermore, an increase in BMI by 1 kg/m^2 and age by 1 year in the

Pediatric Type II Diabetes. https://doi.org/10.1016/B978-0-323-55138-0.00006-1

study participant was associated with 6% and 13% greater risk of developing hypertension, respectively.[17] An earlier study from Arkansas of 50 African American patients with T1D and T2D showed that more than 30% of T2D youth presented with hypertension.[18] In comparison to these studies, Upchurch et al. retrospectively reviewed the records of 98 African American, Hispanic, and other ethnicity Texas adolescents with T2D and found elevated systolic and diastolic blood pressure in about 49% and 11% of their patients, respectively.[19] Although these findings illustrate that similar to adults, hypertension is more common in T2D than T1D in children and adolescents, it is concerning to note that hypertension at diagnosis is eight times more common in T2D compared with T1D.[20]

Despite the common occurrence of hypertension in association with diabetes, it is frequently underdiagnosed. In the general pediatric population, Hansel et al. demonstrated that a diagnosis of hypertension or high blood pressure was made in only 26% of children with hypertension.[21] Of note, only 7.4% of with T1D and 31.9% of T2D in the SEARCH study were aware of their hypertension diagnosis.[15] Hypertension significantly increases cardiovascular risk and predisposes to development of other diabetes comorbidities including stroke, end stage renal disease (ESRD), coronary artery disease (CAD), retinopathy, and amputations. Better understanding of the pathophysiology of hypertension in diabetes will help to formulate improved treatment strategies for these comorbidities.

Pathogenesis

Data from large epidemiological studies have consistently demonstrated that high blood pressure is associated with high BMI.[22,23] Children with obesity have approximately a threefold higher risk for hypertension than nonobese children.[24] A complex interaction of environmental, genetic, vascular, and neurological pathophysiological mechanisms contributes to elevated blood pressures in obesity and T2D (Fig. 6.1).

1. **Environmental Factors:** Alterations in diet seen in obesity including an increase in sodium intake and imbalance in omega 3 and omega 6 fatty acid intake have been cited as possible mechanisms for increased blood pressure seen in obesity.[25] Reduced sodium intake and increased consumption of diets rich in omega 3 fatty acids such as fish oil have been shown to be beneficial in hypertension.[25] These dietary modifications seen in T2D and obesity in conjunction with the changes in gut microbiota likely play a role in mediating the metabolic changes including hypertension.[25]

2. **Genetics:** A few genetic links have been reported to date between hypertension and T2D. Lipin 1 is a phosphatidate phosphatase enzyme that is important for synthesis of diacylglycerol and for adipocyte differentiation.[26] Mutations in LPIN1 gene are linked to metabolic syndrome and T2D.[26] Recently, single nucleotide polymorphisms (SNPs) in this gene have been reported in men with hypertension suggesting a genetic link in predisposition to both

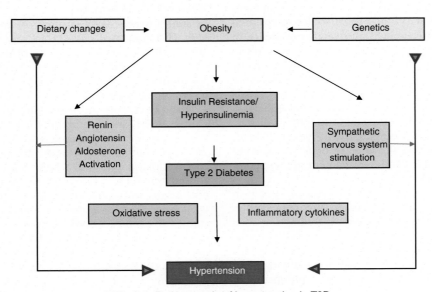

FIG. 6.1 Pathogenesis of hypertension in T2D.

diabetes, obesity and hypertension.[26] Epigenetic changes such as micro RNA modifications are also believed to contribute to hypertension in obesity.[25]

3. Increased expression of **11 β-hydroxy-steroid dehydrogenase** type 1, which is produced in the central abdominal adipocytes, is associated with abdominal obesity. This enzyme catalyzes the conversion of cortisone to cortisol and may be responsible for the hypertension associated with central abdominal fat accumulation.[27]

4. **Dysregulation of renin angiotensin aldosterone system (RAAS)** has been noted in rodents and human with obesity and diabetes.[28,29] Giachetti et al. examined the presence of angiotensinogen in visceral and subcutaneous fat tissue in lean and obese patients. They found that adipose tissue from obese patients expressed angiotensinogen significantly, more so in visceral tissue and correlated significantly with BMI suggesting RAAS activation in obese individuals.[30] Additionally, alterations at the level of the kidney leading to changes in intrarenal RAAS have been suggested.[25,29] Accumulation of perirenal fat may increase the intraarterial pressures and can result in activation of RAAS.[29] Furthermore, it has been hypothesized that there could be local intrarenal angiotensin 2 production in T2D that may account for the observed increase in the renal perfusion rates, despite low renin levels sometimes seen in this condition.[31]

5. **Hyperactivity of the sympathetic nervous system** (SNS) in obese individuals has been consistently recognized as a cause of hypertension.[25] Variability in heart rate and blood pressure with elevated norepinephrine and epinephrine levels are noted in obese children providing evidence for increased sympathetic activity.[24,32] Leptin, the satiety inducing hormone, whose levels are elevated in obesity is considered to mediate this SNS over activity. Leptin stimulates the production of melanocortin (α-melanocyte-stimulating hormone; MSH) that acts through melanocortin receptor 4 (MCR4) to stimulate SNS.[33,34] Other plausible mechanisms for SNS activation in obesity and T2D include RAAS activation and insulin resistance that is described in the following section.

6. **Insulin resistance and hyperinsulinemia:** Several early studies reported positive correlations between insulin levels and elevated blood pressure implicating hyperinsulinemia as a cause of hypertension.[35–38] However, it has been proven that insulin resistance and not hyperinsulinemia regulates blood pressures via various mechanisms. Euglycemic clamp studies have confirmed the presence of insulin resistance in subjects with essential hypertension who do not have diabetes.[39] Insulin resistance influences blood pressure by acting not only on the smooth muscle but also through it actions on the vascular endothelium.[25] Insulin stimulates calcium efflux from vascular smooth muscle (VSM) and decreases smooth muscle responsiveness to vasoconstrictors.[40] Insulin resistance therefore increases VSM calcium resulting in increased VSM tone leading to hypertension.[40] Insulin is also a vasodilatory hormone that regulates the enzyme nitrous oxide (NO) synthase, an enzyme important for NO production through the phosphatidylinositol 3-kinase-dependent (PI3K) pathway.[41,42] Consequently, insulin-resistant states are prone to impaired NO production and increased vascular tone and increased susceptibility to hypertension.[41,42] Furthermore, insulin resistance contributes overexpression of endothelin-1 (a vasoconstrictor) by altering mitogen-activated protein kinase (MAPK)-dependent signaling in vascular endothelium.[42,43]

7. **Oxidative stress** plays a crucial role in mediating high blood pressure in diabetes. The metabolic alterations in diabetes result in increased mitochondrial free radical production in the vascular endothelium. Hyperglycemia-induced mitochondrial superoxides inhibit the endothelial Nitrous Oxide Synthase (NOS) activity thereby resulting in hypertension.[44] Subjects with noninsulin-dependent diabetes have increased arterial stiffness as manifested by an increased aortic pulse wave velocity compared with controls.[45] It has been postulated that glycation products of collagen and elastin and the buildup of advanced glycation end products might contribute to the arterial stiffness and hypertension.[45,46] Obesity is a proinflammatory state characterized by cytokine-mediated vascular and renal injury. Cytotoxic T cells and helper T cells induce vascular injury by increasing proinflammatory mediator IL-17.[47]

Screening, Diagnosis and Management of Hypertension in Diabetes

Hypertension in T2D predisposes to development of cardiovascular, neurological, and renal complications. Early diagnosis and management is important to achieve favorable outcomes. The American Diabetes Association (ADA) recommends screening all patients with T2D for hypertension at every visit.[48] Blood pressure has to be measured with an appropriate size cuff and in the sitting position in the right arm.[9,49] As alluded to earlier, in the pediatric population, blood pressure is plotted against the norms for age, gender, and height.[49] If the first blood pressure obtained at a visit is greater than the 90th percentile, two other measurements using auscultatory method is recommended and the average of the blood pressures is used to categorize hypertension in the child.[9]

Elevated blood pressure predisposes to the development of microalbuminuria and urine albumin excretion has an independent relationship with carotid intima thickness in hypertensive adults with T2D.[50] Subjects with insulin resistance with no diabetes also have microalbuminuria suggesting increased permeability following endothelial injury.[50,51] Therefore, microalbumin is predictor of cardiovascular morbidities and is considered an early screening tool for cardiovascular disease detection.

Management of Hypertension in Diabetes

In children with T2D the initial management of elevated blood pressure greater than the 95th percentile found at least on three occasions is lifestyle modification consisting of weight loss measures and reduced sodium intake.[9,14,49] The upper limit of sodium intake recommended by Institute of Medicine is 1900 mg, for age 4–8 years, 2200 mg for 9–13 years, and 2300 mg for 14–18 years, respectively.[52] If the blood pressure continues to be greater than the 95th percentile after 6 months of lifestyle changes, the first line medication is an angiotensin converting enzyme (ACE) inhibitor.[49] Patients who do not tolerate the ACE inhibitors and develop dry cough, dizziness, or hyperkalemia may be started on angiotensin receptor blockers (ARB).[49] Although it has been recommended that lifestyle modification to be attempted for 6 months, given the poor success with this approach, use of an antihypertensive agent at the same time as initiation of lifestyle change may be reasonable. The primary goal of treatment is to achieve blood pressure reduction. Multiple studies in adults attest to the improved cardiovascular and renal outcomes with medical management of hypertension. In the United Kingdom Prospective Diabetes Study (UKPDS), adults with tight blood pressure control had greater reductions in strokes (44%), microvascular end points (37%), diabetes-related end points (24%), and deaths related to diabetes (32%).[53] A 10-mm Hg reduction in blood pressure was associated with a 12% reduction in diabetes complications and a 15% reduction in diabetes deaths.[54] The Heart Outcomes Prevention Evaluation (HOPE) study showed a significant reduction in cardiovascular complications with the use of ACE inhibitors in adults.[55] In this study, treatment with ACE inhibitors prevented 150 events in 70

patients, when 100 patients with diabetes were treated for 4 years.[55] Early diagnosis and management of underlying hypertension can produce major improvements in clinical care of patients with T2D.

NEPHROPATHY IN T2D

Diabetic nephropathy is defined as the presence of (a) persistent microalbuminuria of 30–300 mg/day or 30–300 mg/g creatinine on a random urine sample, or (b) macroalbuminuria of more than 300 mg/day or 300 mg/g of creatinine in random urine sample or (c) overt nephropathy with decrease in creatinine clearance and persistent decline in estimated glomerular filtration rate.[56] The overall prevalence of nephropathy in youth with diabetes has increased in the last decade[57] and has contributed to morbidity and mortality in diabetes. Youth onset diabetes is particularly associated with increased complications such as nephropathy. In a study of Pima Indians with diabetes, early onset T2D in youth less than 20 years of age was associated with five times higher risk of developing end stage renal disease compared with those who developed diabetes between 20 and 55 years of age.[58] In the SEARCH for Diabetes youth registry, the age adjusted prevalence of nephropathy in youth with T2D was 19.9%.[59] In the TODAY study, microalbuminuria was found in 6.3% at baseline and 16.6% at the end of 4 years of follow-up.[17]

Data from earlier studies had indicated that the risk of renal disease in T1D and T2D were comparable.[60,61] However, more recent data suggest that the burden of renal disease in youth with T2D is higher compared with T1D. In an Australian cohort, 47.4% of T2D youth had microalbuminuria in comparison with 13.1% in T1D despite a shorter duration of diabetes and similar glycemic control.[5] Of note, in this study, there were no differences for renal function that was assessed using glomerular filtration rates. However, a Canadian study showed a fourfold increased risk of renal failure in T2D compared with T1D diabetes in the young T2D.[62] Similar rates were found for renal disease in the SEARCH study with 19.9% for T2D versus 5.8% for T1D.[59] These studies supported the development of complications as early as late adolescence and young adulthood.

PATHOPHYSIOLOGY

Multiple factors in T2D including insulin resistance and hyperglycemia in addition to renal hemodynamic changes contribute to the nephropathy in diabetes (Fig. 6.2). Understanding the pathological changes

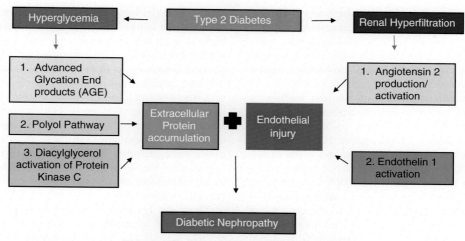

FIG. 6.2 Pathogenesis of nephropathy in T2D.

noted at the renal tissue level provides insight into the mechanisms that lead to these changes. The Renal Pathology Society classifies the changes seen in diabetic nephropathy into four stages[63]

1. Class 1: Glomerular Basement Membrane (GBM) thickening resulting from accumulation of extracellular matrix proteins such as collagen and fibrin in the GBM only.
2. Class 2: Mesangial expansion Mild (2a), Severe (2b) due to extracellular protein accumulation in mesangium in addition to GBM.
3. Class 3: Nodular Sclerosis (Kimmelstein Wilson lesions). These lesions are characterized by mesangial cell lysis and endothelial cell detachment from the GBM in the areas of mesangial matrix accumulation
4. Advanced Diabetic Glomerulosclerosis: This stage is characterized by sclerotic lesions, which represent end products of the protein accumulation in >50% of the glomeruli.

These pathological changes have been studied in detail mainly in the adult population with T2D. Given the small number who develop ESRD among youth with T2D, studies examining the pathology in young adolescents are limited. Sellers and associates reported that 9 out of 10 children who had renal biopsies of the 90 Canadian First Nation children they reviewed had immune complex disease and none had classical diabetes nephropathy findings.[64] Although diabetes is the most common cause of end stage renal disease in older aboriginal adults from Canada, glomerulonephritis and not diabetes has been shown to be the leading cause of renal involvement in children and young adults less than 22 years.[65]

Chronic hyperglycemia is an important reason for the pathological changes seen in diabetic nephropathy. First, hyperglycemia leads to formation of advanced glycation end products (AGE), which accumulates along the vessel wall resulting in renal vascular damage.[66] The receptors for these advance glycated end products (RAGE) are found on many cells including macrophages and endothelial cells. Activation of RAGEs also stimulates production of free radicals and cytokines such as vascular endothelial growth factors (VEGF) transforming growth factor beta (TGF-β), both of which are mediators of renal injury.[67] VEGF produces endothelial injury and VEGF blockade results in improvement of renal function.[68,69]

TGF-β induces mesangial proliferation by inducing epithelial mesangial transition of the tubular epithelial cells.[70] TGF-β, in addition to being stimulated by AGEs, is also directly induced by glucose, angiotensin 2, and endothelin and plays a pivotal role in mediating nephropathy.[67]

A second mechanism by which hyperglycemia contributes to nephropathy is by conversion of glucose to sorbitol through the aldose reductase pathway, one of the enzymatic reactions of the polyol pathway that utilizes nicotinamide adenine dinucleotide phosphate (NADPH).[71] The pentose phosphate pathway gets upregulated secondary to the NADPH reduction leading to protein kinase c activation and subsequent prostaglandin production and loss of mesangial contractility, finally resulting in increased ultrafiltration at glomeruli.[71] Additionally, glucose gets converted to diacylglycerol directly, which then activates protein kinase c resulting in the above-mentioned changes.[71] Finally, the free radicals generated by all of these processes have a potential to induce significant renal vascular injury.[71] As alluded to earlier in the hypertension section, insulin resistance plays a critical role in decreasing the vascular reactivity to vasoactive agents and has been linked to endothelial injury and renal damage.

Renal hyperfiltration is a prominent finding in early stages of kidney injury in diabetes and is the second mechanism contributing to the pathological changes in diabetic nephropathy. Hypertension is a common comorbidity in diabetes and is the dominant factor causing the development of nephropathy. Hypertension may be partly responsible for increasing the increased glomerular pressure; however, increased filtration is noted in diabetes even in the absence of hypertension.[66,72] These changes to the renal vascular dynamics are mediated by hormones such as angiotensin 2 and endothelin.[66,67] Intrarenal angiotensin 2 production has been postulated as a cause of hyperfiltration seen in diabetes.[31] Endothelin 1 is a potent vasoconstrictor, which is overexpressed in hyperglycemia, and in addition to increasing glomerular pressure triggers extracellular matrix changes resulting in mesangial cell expansion.[73]

SCREENING AND MANAGEMENT

The diabetes kidney disease ADA consensus statement has defined the use of two important screening tools for nephropathy in diabetes: (a) estimated glomerular filtration rate (eGFR) as a marker for renal function and (b) microalbuminuria, as an indicator for renal damage.[74] A confirmation of albuminuria should also be obtained in at least two of three samples obtained over a period of 3–6 months.[74] Urine samples should be obtained first thing in the morning, to avoid identification of exercise-induced proteinuria. Hyperfiltration precedes the development of renal impairment in diabetic nephropathy and current eGFR estimations are imprecise at high GFR, which makes it a less effective test.[75] Microalbuminuria assays, on the other hand, can be equally inaccurate and were found to have about 40% variation compared with standard mass spectrometry assays in one study.[76] Furthermore, albuminuria is considerably increased by increase in blood sugars, blood pressures, high protein diet, and with fever and exercise in addition to having significant intraindividual variability daily.[74] Despite these limitations, these tests remain invaluable in detecting early renal involvement in diabetes.

The two main factors that impact renal outcomes in diabetes are as follows: (1) achieving good glycemic control and (b) hypertension management. Monitoring glycemic control with hemoglobin A1C (A1C) is tricky in renal impairment when eGFR starts to decline. With decreasing renal function the RBC life spans get shortened and results in inaccurate A1C values.[74] Furthermore, chronic kidney disease predisposes to anemia, hypoglycemia, and decreased insulin clearance, all of which can lower A1C levels.[74] Other markers such as fructosamine, 1,5 anhydroglucitol, and glycated albumin have been evaluated; of these, glycated albumin offers some promise.[74,77,78] Nevertheless, it is important to monitor blood glucose levels closely and make insulin dosing adjustments to avoid micro- and macrovascular complications.

There are no guidelines specific for nephropathy management in adolescents and youth with diabetes. The Kidney Disease Improving Global Outcomes (KDIGO) group recommends treating blood pressure greater than 90th percentile with antihypertensive to maintain it in the range of 50th percentile for age, gender, and height.[79] It is evident from existing data that inhibition of the RAAS system is the first line of management for diabetic kidney disease.[80] Multiple studies including the UKPDS in adults with T2D have shown that subjects assigned to better blood pressure control using ACE inhibitors had improved albumin excretion and renal function.[53,80,81] However, a study of the effects of ACE inhibitors in youth with T1D demonstrated that although marginally less microalbuminuria could be identified, there was no statistically significant decrease in urinary albumin excretion.[82] This study bears repeating in T2D youth who have a higher prevalence of hypertension.

United States Food and Drug Administration (FDA) approved medications for management for T2D in youth are limited and consist of insulin and metformin. Given the renal excretion of metformin, it has to be used with caution in renal impairment, making T2D management in youth even more challenging.[83] Most data for diabetic nephropathy management come from adult studies due to the small number of patients who develop end stage renal disease in youth and the difficulty in recruiting those patients for drug studies. Nevertheless, the increasing prevalence of T2D and associated renal disease in youth clearly poses huge health risk and dictates further research.

Hypertension and nephropathy were once considered as diabetes comorbidities of middle age. However, with the increased incidence of T2D as a result of the worldwide obesity epidemic, these disorders are now seen in adolescence and young adulthood. Research in this area has provided mechanistic insight into the etiopathogenesis of these comorbidities and has helped to improve outcome in adults. Future studies should be aimed at screening children at risk of comorbidities, and providing effective age appropriate therapeutic strategies.

REFERENCES

1. Ogden CL, Carroll MD, Kit BK, Flegal KM. Prevalence of obesity and trends in body mass index among US children and adolescents, 1999–2010. *JAMA.* 2012;307:483–490.
2. Skinner AC, Skelton JA. Prevalence and trends in obesity and severe obesity among children in the United States, 1999–2012. *JAMA Pediatr.* 2014;168:561–566.
3. Mayer-Davis EJ, Lawrence JM, Dabelea D, et al. Incidence trends of type 1 and type 2 diabetes among youths, 2002–2012. *N Engl J Med.* 2017;376:1419–1429.
4. Dabelea D, Mayer-Davis EJ, Saydah S, et al. Prevalence of type 1 and type 2 diabetes among children and adolescents from 2001 to 2009. *JAMA.* 2014;311:1778–1786.
5. Constantino MI, Molyneaux L, Limacher-Gisler F, et al. Long-term complications and mortality in young-onset diabetes: type 2 diabetes is more hazardous and lethal than type 1 diabetes. *Diabetes Care.* 2013;36:3863–3869.
6. Weiss R, Dziura J, Burgert TS, et al. Obesity and the metabolic syndrome in children and adolescents. *N Engl J Med.* 2004;350:2362–2374.
7. International Diabetes Federation. Metabolic syndrome in children and adolescents. In: *The IDF Consensus.* 007.
8. Cook S, Weitzman M, Auinger P, et al. Prevalence of a metabolic syndrome phenotype in adolescents: findings from the third National Health and Nutrition Examination Survey, 1988-1994. *Arch Pediatr Adolesc Med.* 2003;157:821–827.
9. Flynn JT, Kaelber DC, Baker-Smith CM, et al. Clinical practice guideline for screening and management of high blood pressure in children and adolescents. *Pediatrics.* 2017;140.
10. Theodore RF, Broadbent J, Nagin D, et al. Childhood to early-midlife systolic blood pressure trajectories: early-life predictors, effect modifiers, and adult cardiovascular outcomes. *Hypertension.* 2015;66:1108–1115.
11. Weaver Jr DJ. Hypertension in children and adolescents. *Pediatr Rev.* 2017;38:369–382.
12. Chorin E, Hassidim A, Hartal M, et al. Trends in adolescents obesity and the association between BMI and blood pressure: a cross-sectional study in 714,922 healthy teenagers. *Am J Hypertens.* 2015;28:1157–1163.
13. Landsberg L, Molitch M. Diabetes and hypertension: pathogenesis, prevention and treatment. *Clin Exp Hypertens.* 2004;26:621–628.
14. Chiang J. Hypertension and diabetic kidney disease in children and adolescents. *Diabetes Spectr.* 2015;28: 220–224.
15. Rodriguez BL, Dabelea D, Liese AD, et al. Prevalence and correlates of elevated blood pressure in youth with diabetes mellitus: the SEARCH for diabetes in youth study. *J Pediatr.* 2010;157:245–251.e1.
16. Eppens MC, Craig ME, Cusumano J, et al. Prevalence of diabetes complications in adolescents with type 2 compared with type 1 diabetes. *Diabetes Care.* 2006;29:1300–1306.
17. TODAY. Rapid rise in hypertension and nephropathy in youth with type 2 diabetes: the TODAY clinical trial. *Diabetes Care.* 2013;36:1735–1741.
18. Scott CR, Smith JM, Cradock MM, Pihoker C. Characteristics of youth-onset noninsulin-dependent diabetes mellitus and insulin-dependent diabetes mellitus at diagnosis. *Pediatrics.* 1997;100:84–91.
19. Upchurch SL, Brosnan CA, Meininger JC, et al. Characteristics of 98 children and adolescents diagnosed with type 2 diabetes by their health care provider at initial presentation. *Diabetes Care.* 2003;26:2209.
20. Pinhas-Hamiel O, Zeitler P. Acute and chronic complications of type 2 diabetes mellitus in children and adolescents. *Lancet.* 2007;369:1823–1831.
21. Hansen ML, Gunn PW, Kaelber DC. Underdiagnosis of hypertension in children and adolescents. *JAMA.* 2007;298:874–879.
22. Rosner B, Prineas R, Daniels SR, Loggie J. Blood pressure differences between blacks and whites in relation to body size among US children and adolescents. *Am J Epidemiol.* 2000;151:1007–1019.
23. Freedman DS, Dietz WH, Srinivasan SR, Berenson GS. The relation of overweight to cardiovascular risk factors among children and adolescents: the Bogalusa Heart Study. *Pediatrics.* 1999;103:1175–1182.
24. Sorof JM, Poffenbarger T, Franco K, et al. Isolated systolic hypertension, obesity, and hyperkinetic hemodynamic states in children. *J Pediatr.* 2002;140:660–666.
25. DeMarco VG, Aroor AR, Sowers JR. The pathophysiology of hypertension in patients with obesity. *Nat Rev Endocrinol.* 2014;10:364–376.
26. Ong KL, Leung RY, Wong LY, et al. Association of a polymorphism in the lipin 1 gene with systolic blood pressure in men. *Am J Hypertens.* 2008;21:539–545.
27. Bujalska IJ, Walker EA, Hewison M, Stewart PM. A switch in dehydrogenase to reductase activity of 11 beta-hydroxysteroid dehydrogenase type 1 upon differentiation of human omental adipose stromal cells. *J Clin Endocrinol Metab.* 2002;87:1205–1210.
28. Boustany CM, Bharadwaj K, Daugherty A, et al. Activation of the systemic and adipose renin-angiotensin system in rats with diet-induced obesity and hypertension. *Am J Physiol Regul Integr Comp Physiol.* 2004;287:R943–R949.
29. Sharma AM. Is there a rationale for angiotensin blockade in the management of obesity hypertension? *Hypertension.* 2004;44:12–19.
30. Giacchetti G, Faloia E, Sardu C, et al. Gene expression of angiotensinogen in adipose tissue of obese patients. *Int J Obes Relat Metab Disord.* 2000;24(suppl 2):S142–S143.
31. Price DA, Porter LE, Gordon M, et al. The paradox of the low-renin state in diabetic nephropathy. *J Am Soc Nephrol.* 1999;10:2382–2391.
32. Voors AW, Webber LS, Berenson GS. Resting heart rate and pressure-rate product of children in a total biracial community: the Bogalusa Heart Study. *Am J Epidemiol.* 1982;116:276–286.

33. Greenfield JR, Miller JW, Keogh JM, et al. Modulation of blood pressure by central melanocortinergic pathways. *N Engl J Med.* 2009;360:44–52.

34. Feber J, Ruzicka M, Geier P, Litwin M. Autonomic nervous system dysregulation in pediatric hypertension. *Curr Hypertens Rep.* 2014;16:426.

35. Lucas CP, Estigarribia JA, Darga LL, Reaven GM. Insulin and blood pressure in obesity. *Hypertension.* 1985;7:702–706.

36. Modan M, Halkin H, Almog S, et al. Hyperinsulinemia. A link between hypertension obesity and glucose intolerance. *J Clin Invest.* 1985;75:809–817.

37. Pozzan R, Brandao AA, da Silva SL, Brandao AP. Hyperglycemia, hyperinsulinemia, overweight, and high blood pressure in young adults: the Rio de Janeiro Study. *Hypertension.* 1997;30:650–653.

38. Sorof J, Daniels S. Obesity hypertension in children: a problem of epidemic proportions. *Hypertension.* 2002;40:441–447.

39. Ferrannini E, Buzzigoli G, Bonadonna R, et al. Insulin resistance in essential hypertension. *N Engl J Med.* 1987;317:350–357.

40. Sowers JR, Khoury S, Standley P, et al. Mechanisms of hypertension in diabetes. *Am J Hypertens.* 1991;4:177–182.

41. Baron AD. Hemodynamic actions of insulin. *Am J Physiol.* 1994;267:E187–E202.

42. Fonseca V, Desouza C, Asnani S, Jialal I. Nontraditional risk factors for cardiovascular disease in diabetes. *Endocr Rev.* 2004;25:153–175.

43. Muniyappa R, Sowers JR. Role of insulin resistance in endothelial dysfunction. *Rev Endocr Metab Disord.* 2013;14:5–12.

44. Du XL, Edelstein D, Dimmeler S, et al. Hyperglycemia inhibits endothelial nitric oxide synthase activity by post-translational modification at the Akt site. *J Clin Invest.* 2001;108:1341–1348.

45. Lehmann ED, Riley WA, Clarkson P, Gosling RG. Non-invasive assessment of cardiovascular disease in diabetes mellitus. *Lancet.* 1997;350(suppl 1):SI14–S19.

46. Amar J, Chamontin B, Pelissier M, et al. Influence of glucose metabolism on nycthemeral blood pressure variability in hypertensives with an elevated waist-hip ratio. A link with arterial distensibility. *Am J Hypertens.* 1995;8:426–428.

47. Harrison DG, Marvar PJ, Titze JM. Vascular inflammatory cells in hypertension. *Front Physiol.* 2012;3:128.

48. de Boer IH, Bangalore S, Benetos A, et al. Diabetes and hypertension: a position statement by the American Diabetes Association. *Diabetes Care.* 2017;40:1273–1284.

49. Springer SC, Silverstein J, Copeland K, et al. Management of type 2 diabetes mellitus in children and adolescents. *Pediatrics.* 2013;131:e648–e664.

50. Stehouwer CD, Nauta JJ, Zeldenrust GC, et al. Urinary albumin excretion, cardiovascular disease, and endothelial dysfunction in non-insulin-dependent diabetes mellitus. *Lancet.* 1992;340:319–323.

51. Volpe M. Microalbuminuria screening in patients with hypertension: recommendations for clinical practice. *Int J Clin Pract.* 2008;62:97–108.

52. Association AH. American Heart Association; 2015. https://www.heart.org/-/media/files/about-us/policy-research/fact-sheets/ucm_489742.pdf.

53. UKPDS. Tight blood pressure control and risk of macrovascular and microvascular complications in type 2 diabetes: UKPDS 38. UK Prospective Diabetes Study Group. *BMJ.* 1998;317:703–713.

54. Adler AI, Stratton IM, Neil HA, et al. Association of systolic blood pressure with macrovascular and microvascular complications of type 2 diabetes (UKPDS 36): prospective observational study. *BMJ.* 2000;321:412–419.

55. Yusuf S, Sleight P, Pogue J, et al. Effects of an angiotensin-converting-enzyme inhibitor, ramipril, on cardiovascular events in high-risk patients. *N Engl J Med.* 2000;342:145–153.

56. Gross JL, de Azevedo MJ, Silveiro SP, et al. Diabetic nephropathy: diagnosis, prevention, and treatment. *Diabetes Care.* 2005;28:164–176.

57. Li L, Jick S, Breitenstein S, Michel A. Prevalence of diabetes and diabetic nephropathy in a large U.S. commercially insured pediatric population, 2002–2013. *Diabetes Care.* 2016;39:278–284.

58. Pavkov ME, Bennett PH, Knowler WC, et al. Effect of youth-onset type 2 diabetes mellitus on incidence of end-stage renal disease and mortality in young and middle-aged Pima Indians. *JAMA.* 2006;296:421–426.

59. Dabelea D, Stafford JM, Mayer-Davis EJ, et al. Association of type 1 diabetes vs type 2 diabetes diagnosed during childhood and adolescence with complications during teenage years and young adulthood. *JAMA.* 2017;317:825–835.

60. Cowie CC, Port FK, Wolfe RA, et al. Disparities in incidence of diabetic end-stage renal disease according to race and type of diabetes. *N Engl J Med.* 1989;321:1074–1079.

61. Ritz E, Stefanski A. Diabetic nephropathy in type II diabetes. *Am J Kidney Dis.* 1996;27:167–194.

62. Dart AB, Sellers EA, Martens PJ, et al. High burden of kidney disease in youth-onset type 2 diabetes. *Diabetes Care.* 2012;35:1265–1271.

63. Tervaert TW, Mooyaart AL, Amann K, et al. Pathologic classification of diabetic nephropathy. *J Am Soc Nephrol.* 2010;21:556–563.

64. Sellers EA, Blydt-Hansen TD, Dean HJ, et al. Macroalbuminuria and renal pathology in First Nation youth with type 2 diabetes. *Diabetes Care.* 2009;32:786–790.

65. Samuel SM, Foster BJ, Hemmelgarn BR, et al. Incidence and causes of end-stage renal disease among Aboriginal children and young adults. *CMAJ.* 2012;184:E758–E764.

66. Cooper ME. Pathogenesis, prevention, and treatment of diabetic nephropathy. *Lancet.* 1998;352:213–219.

67. Soldatos G, Cooper ME. Diabetic nephropathy: important pathophysiologic mechanisms. *Diabetes Res Clin Pract.* 2008;82(suppl 1):S75–S79.

68. Hohenstein B, Hausknecht B, Boehmer K, et al. Local VEGF activity but not VEGF expression is tightly regulated during diabetic nephropathy in man. *Kidney Int.* 2006;69:1654–1661.

69. de Vriese AS, Tilton RG, Elger M, et al. Antibodies against vascular endothelial growth factor improve early renal dysfunction in experimental diabetes. *J Am Soc Nephrol.* 2001;12:993–1000.

70. Lan HY. Tubular epithelial-myofibroblast transdifferentiation mechanisms in proximal tubule cells. *Curr Opin Nephrol Hypertens.* 2003;12:25–29.

71. Dunlop M. Aldose reductase and the role of the polyol pathway in diabetic nephropathy. *Kidney Int Suppl.* 2000;77:S3–S12.

72. Ohara N, Hanyu O, Hirayama S, et al. Hypertension increases urinary excretion of immunoglobulin G, ceruloplasmin and transferrin in normoalbuminuric patients with type 2 diabetes mellitus. *J Hypertens.* 2014;32: 432–438.

73. Hargrove GM, Dufresne J, Whiteside C, et al. Diabetes mellitus increases endothelin-1 gene transcription in rat kidney. *Kidney Int.* 2000;58:1534–1545.

74. Tuttle KR, Bakris GL, Bilous RW, et al. Diabetic kidney disease: a report from an ADA Consensus Conference. *Diabetes Care.* 2014;37:2864–2883.

75. Magee GM, Bilous RW, Cardwell CR, et al. Is hyperfiltration associated with the future risk of developing diabetic nephropathy? A meta-analysis. *Diabetologia.* 2009;52: 691–697.

76. Bachmann LM, Nilsson G, Bruns DE, et al. State of the art for measurement of urine albumin: comparison of routine measurement procedures to isotope dilution tandem mass spectrometry. *Clin Chem.* 2014;60:471–480.

77. Freedman BI, Andries L, Shihabi ZK, et al. Glycated albumin and risk of death and hospitalizations in diabetic dialysis patients. *Clin J Am Soc Nephrol.* 2011;6:1635–1643.

78. Kim WJ, Park CY, Lee KB, et al. Serum 1,5-anhydroglucitol concentrations are a reliable index of glycemic control in type 2 diabetes with mild or moderate renal dysfunction. *Diabetes Care.* 2012;35:281–286.

79. KDIGO. http://www.kdigo.org/clinical_practice_guidelines/pdf/CKD/KDIGO_2012_CKD_GL.pdf.

80. Lewis EJ, Hunsicker LG, Clarke WR, et al. Renoprotective effect of the angiotensin-receptor antagonist irbesartan in patients with nephropathy due to type 2 diabetes. *N Engl J Med.* 2001;345:851–860.

81. Ravid M, Savin H, Jutrin I, et al. Long-term effect of ACE inhibition on development of nephropathy in diabetes mellitus type II. *Kidney Int Suppl.* 1994;45:S161–S164.

82. Marcovecchio ML, Chiesa ST, Bond S, et al. ACE inhibitors and statins in adolescents with type 1 diabetes. *N Engl J Med.* 2017;377:1733–1745.

83. Heaf J. Metformin in chronic kidney disease: time for a rethink. *Perit Dial Int.* 2014;34:353–357.

Dyslipidemia and Type II Diabetes

LORRAINE KATZ, MD • BRETT BARRETT, DO, MS

INTRODUCTION

As the rate of childhood obesity has risen over the past few decades, so has the incidence of children and adolescents diagnosed with type 2 diabetes. The SEARCH for Diabetes in Youth study, a cross-sectional, population based study conducted across six centers, estimated a prevalence of type 2 diabetes in youth of 0.46 per 1000 in 2009.[1] The high prevalence of obesity in youth has also led to an increase in type 2 diabetes and dyslipidemia.[2] Recognizing diabetes early in its course is imperative in managing complications that are associated with this disease, including dyslipidemia.

DIABETES AND DYSLIPIDEMIA

Dyslipidemia is defined as a lipoprotein disorder promoting the development of atherosclerosis. The lipid abnormalities included in this definition are increased low-density lipoprotein cholesterol, decreased high-density lipoprotein cholesterol, and increased serum triglycerides. Lipid abnormalities have been strongly linked to the risk of cardiovascular disease (CVD) in diabetes in adults, but is less understood in youth. Data in adults with diabetes have shown that lipoprotein composition is more atherogenic and is influenced by glycemic control. The majority of research done on the subject of dyslipidemia in diabetes in youth and has been performed in type 1 diabetes. The SEARCH for Diabetes in Youth study revealed that a large proportion of youth aged 10–22 with type 1 diabetes had lipid concentrations greater than the recommended targets[3] and that mean lipid levels and presence of dyslipidemia are influenced by glycemic control. Children with poor glycemic control and type 1 diabetes have higher prevalence of dyslipidemia, specifically total cholesterol, LDL cholesterol, and non-HDL cholesterol than nondiabetic youth. SEARCH data showed that regardless of glycemic control, children with type 1 diabetes have significantly elevated apoB levels and have more small dense LDL particles than nondiabetic children.[4]

TYPE 2 DIABETES AND DYSLIPIDEMIA IN CHILDREN

It is known that in both adults and children with type 2 diabetes, the combination of obesity, insulin resistance, and relative insulin deficiency is associated with elevated serum triglycerides, decreased HDL cholesterol, and higher LDL cholesterol. Dyslipidemia is very common in adults with type 2 diabetes, and we now know that a substantial portion of children with type 2 diabetes have dyslipidemia. The SEARCH for Diabetes in Youth study showed that 33% of youth with type 2D had total cholesterol greater than 200 mg/dL; 24% had LDL cholesterol greater than 130 mg/dL; 29% had triglyceride concentration greater than 150 mg/dL; and 44% had HDL cholesterol level less than 40 mg/dL.[3]

The Treatment Options for type 2 Diabetes in Adolescents and Youth (TODAY) study was designed to assess the effect of diabetes treatment on duration of metabolic control. This study included 699 multiethnic participants aged 10–17 years diagnosed with type 2 diabetes for less than 2 years. The youth were randomized to three possible groups: metformin, metformin plus rosiglitazone, or metformin plus lifestyle changes. Statins were initiated for LDL cholesterol greater than 130 mg/dL or triglycerides greater than or equal to 300 mg/dL. Studies have shown in adults with diabetes that statin therapy has been beneficial to dyslipidemia,[5,6] but specific benefit in children with type 2 diabetes has not yet been demonstrated. The TODAY study showed that LDL cholesterol increased with increasing HbA1c. After 36 months of follow-up, the prevalence of elevated LDL cholesterol or those on lipid lowering therapy increased to 10.7%. Elevated triglycerides at baseline were seen in 21% and this increased to 23.3% after the 36 months of follow-up. Treatment assignment had no significant effect on LDL or non-HDL cholesterol. However, triglycerides were lower in the metformin plus lifestyle group than metformin alone. Metformin plus lifestyle also attenuated the negative effect of elevated hemoglobin A1C levels on triglyceride levels in all patients and on HDL cholesterol levels in female patients.[7]

Pediatric Type II Diabetes. https://doi.org/10.1016/B978-0-323-55138-0.00007-3

Further analysis from the TODAY study attempted to determine the impact of insulin therapy on lipid and inflammatory markers in youth who had reached primary outcome. This study subgroup included the 285 participants who failed to sustain glycemic control on randomized treatment (primary outcome: HbA1c >8%) and 363 who were compared with those who maintained glycemic control. Upon failing to maintain control, insulin therapy was started. Of note, in those patients who had LDL cholesterol >130 mg/dL, statin therapy was initiated. Changes in lipids and inflammatory markers were then measured over time. The results revealed again that progression of dyslipidemia was related to glycemic control. In the primary outcome group, insulin therapy had a modest impact of HbA1c, and decreased the rise in total cholesterol, LDL cholesterol, and total apolipoprotein B. Statin use in this group also increased from 8.6% to 22% one year after reaching primary outcome. The increase in triglycerides and nonesterified free fatty acids stabilized after initiation of insulin, independent of HbA1c. The analysis showed that insulin therapy without improvement of glycemic control showed little benefit.[8] As expected, glycemic control among adolescents with type 2 diabetes is often poor. Studies have reported that less than half of adolescents with type 2 diabetes regularly attend follow-up visits.[9] A study in Canadian patients reported an average hemoglobin A1C concentration of 12%, even among patients who are actively following up in clinic.[10] As it has been established that diabetes is a major risk factor for cardiovascular disease,[11] given the poor control and follow-up for T2D in this age group, it is important to take preventative measures for dyslipidemia and related comorbidities.

It is well known that obese children can have type 2 diabetes along with metabolic, syndrome, and liver disease. Clinical effects of obesity can be seen as early as infancy.[12] There is significant overlap with T2 diabetes and metabolic syndrome, as well as with fatty liver disease given the role insulin may play in both diseases. Nonalcoholic fatty liver disease NAFLD is more common in children with metabolic syndrome. A recent study of 254 children aged 6–17 years with nonalcoholic fatty liver disease showed that 26% met criteria for metabolic syndrome.[13] As lipogenesis and lipolysis in the liver are influenced by insulin, it is likely that the hyperinsulinemia due to insulin resistance is etiologic.[14]

The potential of NAFLD comorbidity with metabolic syndrome is common. The most widely accepted theory of nonalcoholic steatohepatitis (NASH) pathogenesis is that of the two-hit hypothesis in which the primary abnormality, accumulation of triglyceride within hepatocytes, occurs due to insulin resistance. Insulin resistance leads to hyperinsulinemia, which in turn promotes de novo hepatic lipogenesis through upregulation of transcription

factors, and an influx of free fatty acids to the liver due to loss of insulin-mediated suppression of lipolysis. Hepatic export of triglycerides as very low-density lipoprotein is also impaired. Following this hepatocellular triglyceride accumulation, the steatotic liver is then vulnerable to a second hit. Proposed sources of this secondary injury include oxidative stress and adipocytokines.[13]

Children with NAFLD have increased prevalence of risk factors for CVD including elevated low-density lipoprotein, increased total cholesterol, and decreased high-density lipoprotein, when compared to matched controls.[15] The severity of NASH, as assessed by the NAFLD activity score is associated with increased triglyceride/HDL, total cholesterol/HDL, and LDL/HDL ratios.[16] Children with NAFLD also have greater carotid arterial intima-media thickness, when compared to obese children without NAFLD.[17] In a study by Corey et al., the resolution of NASH in children was associated with a significant decrease in total cholesterol levels from baseline compared to those who did not experience a resolution of NASH (mean change –10.0 mg/dL vs. –0.9 mg/dL). In addition, in those whose NASH had resolved, there was a significant decrease in non-HDL cholesterol levels compared to subjects without resolution of NASH (mean change –7.3 mg/dL vs. 1.1).[1,8]

SCREENING FOR DYSLIPIDEMIA

Children with low A1C levels and type 1 diabetes have lipid profiles that are similar to or even less atherogenic than those observed in nondiabetic youth. Based upon observations from adult trials, the American Diabetes Association in combination with the American Academy of Pediatrics developed guidelines for dyslipidemia screening and treatment in children with both type 1 and type 2 diabetes.[19] The ADA 2017 recommendations in patients with type 1 diabetes above age 10 is for a fasting lipid panel to be obtained shortly after diagnosis, but after glycemic control is established. This should include total cholesterol, LDL cholesterol, HDL cholesterol, and triglycerides. Goal levels of LDL cholesterol are less than 100 mg/dL; for HDL cholesterol, goals are greater than 35 mg/dL; and for triglycerides, goals are less than 150 mg/dL. If levels are abnormal, annual monitoring is recommended. If LDL cholesterol level is less than 100 mg/dL, repeating every 3–5 years is reasonable. In those with type 2 diabetes, pediatric patients should be screened after glycemic control is achieved regardless of age. After screening, the same goals as for type 1 diabetic patients are followed (Fig. 7.1).[20]

TREATMENT OF DYSLIPIDEMIA

Initial treatment for dyslipidemia in youth consists of optimizing glucose control and medical nutrition

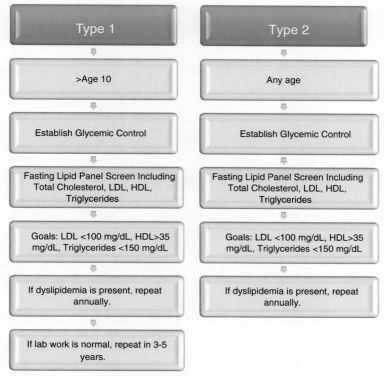

FIG. 7.1 Screening for dyslipidemia in children with diabetes.[20]

therapy to decrease the amount of saturated fat in the diet. Specifically the American Heart Association step 2 diet is suggested. This diet recommends daily dietary cholesterol intake of less than 200 mg per day and saturated fat of less than 7% of all total calories (Fig. 7.2). Follow-up of fasting lipids should be obtained at 3 months and again at 6 months after diet and lifestyle changes have been implemented. After age 10 years, the addition of a statin is suggested in patients who despite lifestyle and nutritional changes, continue to have LDL-cholesterol level greater than 160 mg/dL or LDL cholesterol greater than 130 mg/dL plus one or more cardiovascular risk factor. Of note, studies in youth have shown short-term safety equivalent to that seen in adults and efficacy in lowering LDL cholesterol levels.[21] However, published data are lacking in long-term efficacy in youth with type 2 diabetes. The goal of medical therapy is an LDL cholesterol value less than 100 mg/dL.[20]

It is important to consider the risks of starting any medication, including statins. In randomized trials, statin therapy seems to cause only slight increase in risk of side effects compared with placebo, and no increased risk of discontinuation of therapy compared with placebo.[22,23] Hepatic dysfunction is one of the more common side effects noted during statin therapy. Clinical studies of statins have demonstrated a 0.5%–3.0% occurrence of persistent elevation in aminotransferases in those receiving statins. This primarily occurred during the first three months of therapy and was dose-dependent. However, several randomized trials have also reported no significant difference in the incidence of persistently elevated aminotransferases between statin and placebo therapy.[24,25] In 2012, the US Food and Drug Administration (FDA) revised its recommendations on statins to only check liver function testing prior to initiation of statin therapy and to only repeat testing for clinical indications.[26]

Statin muscle-related adverse events are fairly uncommon. Myalgias and myopathy occur with the highest frequency at 2%–10% based on the literature.[27-29] However, severe myonecrosis and clinical rhabdomyolysis are much rarer (0.5% and less than 0.1%, respectively). Increased susceptibility to statin-associated myopathy occurs in patients with hypothyroidism, acute or chronic renal failure, and obstructive

Nutrient*	Recommended Intake as Percent of Total Calories	
	Step I Diet	Step II Diet
Total Fat	30% or less	30% or less
Saturated	7 - 10%	less than 7%
Polyunsaturated	Up to 10%	Up to 10%
Monounsaturated	Up to 15%	Up to 15%
Carbohydrate	55% or more	55% or more
Protein	Approximately 15%	Approximately 15%
Cholesterol	Less than 300 mg per day	Less than 200 mg per day
Total Calories	To achieve and maintain desired weight	To achieve and maintain desired weight

FIG. 7.2 American Heart Association step I and step II diets.[20]

liver disease. Hypothyroidism is also known to be a cause of dyslipidemia and therefore would be a consideration for screening prior to statin therapy initiation.[30]

There has been concern of renal dysfunction with statin use; however, the significance of renal injury and the statin being the cause of injury have been questioned. Statins appear to be able to cause proteinuria through tubular inhibition of active transport of small molecular weight proteins.[31] There have been reports to the FDA about proteinuria with statin use as well. However, the FDA has stated that this is benign finding.[32]

Elevated triglycerides with levels between 150 and 699 mg/dL should be managed by maximizing glucose control and weight loss. In those patients with triglyceride levels greater than 1000 mg/dL, treatment should be considered with fibric acid or niacin due to the risk for pancreatitis.[33] Fibric acid derivatives are most commonly used for treating severe hypertriglyceridemia in children due to side effects of niacin such as flushing, abdominal pain, vomiting, headache, or elevated serum aminotransferase levels.[34] Fibric acid agents raise high-density lipoprotein cholesterol (HDL-C) and lower TG levels.[35] Again, there is not sufficient data in pediatric patients with type 2 diabetes for clear recommendations.

Omega-3 fatty acids have long been known to lower plasma triglycerides.[36] Although the triglyceride lowering due to fish oils are not evident at intakes in the normal Western diet[37] they manifest at pharmaceutical doses (i.e., >3 g/day of EPA + DHA).[38] The pharmaceutical grade product of omega-3 acid fatty acids provides EPA and DHA as acid ethyl esters, and the approved dose is 4, 1-g capsules per day that provides 1860 mg of EPA and 1500 mg of DHA for a total of 3.4 g omega-3 fatty acids per day. The triglyceride lowering effect of 3–4 g per day of omega-3 fatty acids has been shown to decrease plasma triglycerides by about 30%.[39]

TYPE 2 DIABETES AND CARDIOVASCULAR RISK

For nearly 70 years, there has been a postulated link between impaired glucose metabolism and atherosclerotic cardiovascular disease. The clustering of risk factors (obesity, insulin resistance, hypertension, and dyslipidemia) now known as metabolic syndrome has been shown to predict higher cardiovascular morbidity, mortality, and risk for diabetes in adults.[40] Features of metabolic syndrome are present in children as well. However, the precise definition has been a matter of debate. In 2007, the International Diabetes Federation attempted a definition of pediatric metabolic syndrome using age-specific diagnostic criteria and proposed that metabolic syndrome to be considered in children aged 6–10 years who are obese (defined as waist circumference (WC) ≥90th percentile) and have other relevant risk factors (such as family history of cardiometabolic disease, which includes myocardial infarction or stroke < age 55) and in children aged 10–16 years who are obese (defined as WC ≥ 90th percentile) and meet the adult metabolic syndrome criteria for triglycerides, HDL-cholesterol, blood pressure, and glucose concentrations.[41] In terms of glucose metabolism, a study has shown that in patients aged 6–16 years, those with fasting blood glucose greater than 100 mg/dL, there was a higher risk of aggregation of hypertension, hypercholesterolemia, and abnormal glycemia.[42]

Central adiposity is an important factor in metabolic syndrome. Weiss et al. showed that obese children with impaired glucose tolerance had different fat distribution than equally obese children who had normal glucose tolerance. The impaired glucose tolerance group had more visceral and intramyocellular fat as opposed to subcutaneous fat.[43] It has been shown that when lipid accumulates in the liver and muscle, the lipid metabolites can cause defects in insulin signaling.[44] Visceral fat has also been shown to secrete higher amounts of inflammatory adipokines, which may be a part of the underlying pathogenesis and morbidity of metabolic syndrome.[45]

Previous studies in adults with type 2 diabetes have established that diabetes is an independent risk factor for cardiovascular disease. The Framingham cardiovascular risk assessment states that type 2 diabetes is equivalent to an increase in age of 10 years in adults. When combined with other risk factors, such as dyslipidemia, type 2 diabetes increases the risk of cardiovascular disease by an additional three- to fourfold greater than that predicted for each risk factor independently.[46]

Children and adolescents with type 2 diabetes are also at increased risk for associated comorbidities including hypertension, dyslipidemia, and nonalcoholic fatty liver disease. Type 2 diabetes, smoking, hypertension, and dyslipidemia are also risks for macrovascular complications. This has been established in adults, but accumulating data suggest that it is also the case for children and adolescents with T2DM.[47] Indicators of atherosclerosis are already present in youth populations with type 2 diabetes and dyslipidemia.[48] Both elevated HbA1c and dyslipidemia can worsen markers of subclinical atherosclerosis in youth with type 2 diabetes, including carotid intima media thickness and arterial stiffness.[49-52] In youth without diabetes, dyslipidemia similar to that of type 2 diabetes is associated with increased indicators of subclinical atherosclerosis over time.[53]

As a secondary aim, TODAY study looked at arterial stiffness in young adults with youth onset type 2 diabetes by measuring femoral, radial, and pedal pulse wave velocity, augmentation index, and brachial distensibility. These measures were compared to published data for obese and lean controls. The report showed that patients with type 2 diabetes had significantly higher arterial stiffness compared with lean and obese controls.[54]

CONCLUSIONS

The epidemic of type 2 diabetes now involves youth. Worsening dyslipidemia over time raises concern for premature development of atherosclerosis in youth

with type 2 diabetes. The challenges in achieving optimal control in adolescents with type 2 diabetes highlight the critical need to promote a healthy lifestyle to prevent or postpone the development of type 2 diabetes as well as its comorbidities. For individuals already found to have early-onset type 2 diabetes, glycemic control must be carefully monitored and treated, adding insulin when necessary.

With regards to type 2 diabetes in the youth, worsening dyslipidemia over time raises concern for premature development of atherosclerosis. In the absence of glycemic control, insulin therapy in the TODAY trial did not improve dyslipidemia. This highlights the importance of optimizing glycemic control to limit comorbidities and improve long-term outcomes of dyslipidemia in youth with T2D. Ongoing monitoring and treatment for diabetes comorbidities, cardiovascular risk factors, and complications are essential to prevent early morbidity and mortality.

REFERENCES

1. Dabelea D, Mayer-Davis EJ, Saydah S, et al. Prevalence of type 1 and type 2 diabetes among children and adolescents from 2001 to 2009. *JAMA*. 2014;311(17):1778–1786.
2. Freedman DS, Mei Z, Srinivasan SR, Berenson GS, Dietz WH. Cardiovascular risk factors and excess adiposity among overweight children and adolescents: the Bogalusa Heart Study. *J Pediatr*. 2007;150(1): 12–17.e12.
3. Kershnar AK, Daniels SR, Imperatore G, et al. Lipid abnormalities are prevalent in youth with type 1 and type 2 diabetes: the SEARCH for diabetes in youth study. *J Pediatr*. 2006;149(3):314–319.
4. Guy J, Ogden L, Wadwa RP, et al. Lipid and lipoprotein profiles in youth with and without type 1 diabetes: the SEARCH for Diabetes in Youth case-control study. *Diabetes Care*. 2009;32(3):416–420.
5. Colhoun HM, Betteridge DJ, Durrington PN, et al. Primary prevention of cardiovascular disease with atorvastatin in type 2 diabetes in the Collaborative Atorvastatin Diabetes Study (CARDS): multicentre randomised placebo-controlled trial. *Lancet*. 2004;364(9435):685–696.
6. Sacks FM, Tonkin AM, Craven T, et al. Coronary heart disease in patients with low LDL-cholesterol: benefit of pravastatin in diabetics and enhanced role for HDL-cholesterol and triglycerides as risk factors. *Circulation*. 2002;105(12):1424–1428.
7. Lipid and inflammatory cardiovascular risk worsens over 3 years in youth with type 2 diabetes: the TODAY clinical trial. *Diabetes Care*. 2013;36(6):1758–1764.
8. Katz L., Bacha F.S.. Gidding S., et al. Changes in Lipid Profiles and Inflammatory Markers in Response to Insulin Therapy in Youth with Type 2 Diabetes (T2D) in the TODAY Trial. 632014.

9. Pinhas-Hamiel O, Zeitler P. Acute and chronic complications of type 2 diabetes mellitus in children and adolescents. *Lancet.* 2007;369(9575):1823–1831.
10. Dean H. Niddm-Y in first nation children in Canada. *Clin Pediatr (Phila).* 1998;37(2):89–96.
11. Grundy SM, D'Agostino Sr RB, Mosca L, et al. Cardiovascular risk assessment based on US cohort studies: findings from a National Heart, Lung, and Blood institute workshop. *Circulation.* 2001;104(4):491–496.
12. Shibli R, Rubin L, Akons H, Shaoul R. Morbidity of overweight (>or=85th percentile) in the first 2 years of life. *Pediatrics.* 2008;122(2):267–272.
13. Patton HM, Yates K, Unalp-Arida A, et al. Association between metabolic syndrome and liver histology among children with nonalcoholic Fatty liver disease. *Am J Gastroenterol.* 2010;105(9):2093–2102.
14. Weiss R. Fat distribution and storage: how much, where, and how. *Eur J Endocrinol.* 2007;157(suppl 1):S39–S45.
15. Schwimmer JB, Pardee PE, Lavine JE, Blumkin AK, Cook S. Cardiovascular risk factors and the metabolic syndrome in pediatric nonalcoholic fatty liver disease. *Circulation.* 2008;118(3):277–283.
16. Nobili V, Alkhouri N, Bartuli A, et al. Severity of liver injury and atherogenic lipid profile in children with nonalcoholic fatty liver disease. *Pediatr Res.* 2010;67(6):665–670.
17. Demircioglu F, Kocyigit A, Arslan N, Cakmakci H, Hizli S, Sedat AT. Intima-media thickness of carotid artery and susceptibility to atherosclerosis in obese children with nonalcoholic fatty liver disease. *J Pediatr Gastroenterol Nutr.* 2008;47(1):68–75.
18. Corey KE, Vuppalanchi R, Vos M, et al. Improvement in liver histology is associated with reduction in dyslipidemia in children with nonalcoholic fatty liver disease. *J Pediatr Gastroenterol Nutr.* 2015;60(3):360–367.
19. Management of dyslipidemia in children and adolescents with diabetes. *Diabetes Care.* 2003;26(7):2194–2197.
20. 12. Children and adolescents. *Diabetes Care.* 2017;40(suppl 1):S105–S113.
21. McCrindle BW, Ose L, Marais AD. Efficacy and safety of atorvastatin in children and adolescents with familial hypercholesterolemia or severe hyperlipidemia: a multicenter, randomized, placebo-controlled trial. *J Pediatr.* 2003;143(1):74–80.
22. Kashani A, Phillips CO, Foody JM, et al. Risks associated with statin therapy: a systematic overview of randomized clinical trials. *Circulation.* 2006;114(25):2788–2797.
23. Armitage J. The safety of statins in clinical practice. *Lancet.* 2007;370(9601):1781–1790.
24. Downs JR, Clearfield M, Weis S, et al. Primary prevention of acute coronary events with lovastatin in men and women with average cholesterol levels: results of AFCAPS/TexCAPS. Air Force/Texas coronary atherosclerosis prevention study. *JAMA.* 1998;279(20):1615–1622.
25. MRC/BHF Heart Protection Study of cholesterol lowering with simvastatin in 20,536 high-risk individuals: a randomised placebo-controlled trial. *Lancet.* 2002;360(9326):7–22.
26. Statin label changes. *Med Lett Drugs Ther.* 2012;54(1386):21.
27. Tobert JA. Efficacy and long-term adverse effect pattern of lovastatin. *Am J Cardiol.* 1988;62(15):28J–34J.
28. Dujovne CA, Chremos AN, Pool JL, et al. Expanded clinical evaluation of lovastatin (EXCEL) study results: IV. Additional perspectives on the tolerability of lovastatin. *Am J Med.* 1991;91(1B):25S–30S.
29. Ganga HV, Slim HB, Thompson PD. A systematic review of statin-induced muscle problems in clinical trials. *Am Heart J.* 2014;168(1):6–15.
30. Lando HM, Burman KD. Two cases of statin-induced myopathy caused by induced hypothyroidism. *Endocr Pract.* 2008;14(6):726–731.
31. Sidaway JE, Davidson RG, McTaggart F, et al. Inhibitors of 3-hydroxy-3-methylglutaryl-CoA reductase reduce receptor-mediated endocytosis in opossum kidney cells. *J Am Soc Nephrol.* 2004;15(9):2258–2265.
32. Grundy SM. The issue of statin safety: where do we stand? *Circulation.* 2005;111(23):3016–3019.
33. Springer SC, Silverstein J, Copeland K, et al. Management of type 2 diabetes mellitus in children and adolescents. *Pediatrics.* 2013;131(2):e648–e664.
34. Colletti RB, Neufeld EJ, Roff NK, McAuliffe TL, Baker AL, Newburger JW. Niacin treatment of hypercholesterolemia in children. *Pediatrics.* 1993;92(1):78–82.
35. Expert panel on integrated guidelines for cardiovascular health and risk reduction in children and adolescents: summary report. *Pediatrics.* 2011;128(suppl 5):S213–S256.
36. Imaichi K, Michaels GD, Gunning B, Grasso S, Fukayama G, Kinsell LW. Studies with the use of fish oil fractions in human subjects. *Am J Clin Nutr.* 1963;13:158–168.
37. Skulas-Ray AC, Kris-Etherton PM, Harris WS, Vanden Heuvel JP, Wagner PR, West SG. Dose-response effects of omega-3 fatty acids on triglycerides, inflammation, and endothelial function in healthy persons with moderate hypertriglyceridemia. *Am J Clin Nutr.* 2011;93(2):243–252.
38. Mori TA, Woodman RJ. The independent effects of eicosapentaenoic acid and docosahexaenoic acid on cardiovascular risk factors in humans. *Curr Opin Clin Nutr Metab Care.* 2006;9(2):95–104.
39. Harris WS, Miller M, Tighe AP, Davidson MH, Schaefer EJ. Omega-3 fatty acids and coronary heart disease risk: clinical and mechanistic perspectives. *Atherosclerosis.* 2008;197(1):12–24.
40. Ford ES. Risks for all-cause mortality, cardiovascular disease, and diabetes associated with the metabolic syndrome: a summary of the evidence. *Diabetes Care.* 2005;28(7):1769–1778.
41. Zimmet P, Alberti G, Kaufman F, et al. The metabolic syndrome in children and adolescents. *Lancet.* 2007;369(9579):2059–2061.
42. Li HY, Wei JN, Ma WY, et al. Hypertension and hypercholesterolemia aggregate in nondiabetic children and adolescents with higher fasting plasma glucose levels. *Pediatr Diabetes.* 2011;12(1):41–49.

CHAPTER 7 Dyslipidemia and Type II Diabetes   **53**

43. Weiss R, Dufour S, Taksali SE, et al. Prediabetes in obese youth: a syndrome of impaired glucose tolerance, severe insulin resistance, and altered myocellular and abdominal fat partitioning. *Lancet.* 2003;362(9388):951–957.

44. Morino K, Petersen KF, Shulman GI. Molecular mechanisms of insulin resistance in humans and their potential links with mitochondrial dysfunction. *Diabetes.* 2006;55(suppl 2):S9–S15.

45. Fain JN, Madan AK, Hiler ML, Cheema P, Bahouth SW. Comparison of the release of adipokines by adipose tissue, adipose tissue matrix, and adipocytes from visceral and subcutaneous abdominal adipose tissues of obese humans. *Endocrinology.* 2004;145(5):2273–2282.

46. Wilson PW, D'Agostino RB, Levy D, Belanger AM, Silbershatz H, Kannel WB. Prediction of coronary heart disease using risk factor categories. *Circulation.* 1998;97(18):1837–1847.

47. Copeland KC, Zeitler P, Geffner M, et al. Characteristics of adolescents and youth with recent-onset type 2 diabetes: the TODAY cohort at baseline. *J Clin Endocrinol Metab.* 2011;96(1):159–167.

48. McGill Jr HC, McMahan CA, Malcom GT, Oalmann MC, Strong JP. Relation of glycohemoglobin and adiposity to atherosclerosis in youth. Pathobiological determinants of atherosclerosis in youth (PDAY) research group. *Arterioscler Thromb Vasc Biol.* 1995;15(4):431–440.

49. Maahs DM, Daniels SR, de Ferranti SD, et al. Cardiovascular disease risk factors in youth with diabetes mellitus: a scientific statement from the American Heart Association. *Circulation.* 2014;130(17):1532–1558.

50. Shah AS, Urbina EM, Khoury PR, Kimball TR, Dolan LM. Lipids and lipoprotein ratios: contribution to carotid intima media thickness in adolescents and young adults with type 2 diabetes mellitus. *J Clin Lipidol.* 2013;7(5):441–445.

51. Urbina EM, Kimball TR, Khoury PR, Daniels SR, Dolan LM. Increased arterial stiffness is found in adolescents with obesity or obesity-related type 2 diabetes mellitus. *J Hypertens.* 2010;28(8):1692–1698.

52. Shah AS, Dolan LM, Kimball TR, et al. Influence of duration of diabetes, glycemic control, and traditional cardiovascular risk factors on early atherosclerotic vascular changes in adolescents and young adults with type 2 diabetes mellitus. *J Clin Endocrinol Metab.* 2009;94(10):3740–3745.

53. Magnussen CG, Venn A, Thomson R, et al. The association of pediatric low- and high-density lipoprotein cholesterol dyslipidemia classifications and change in dyslipidemia status with carotid intima-media thickness in adulthood evidence from the cardiovascular risk in Young Finns study, the Bogalusa Heart study, and the CDAH (Childhood Determinants of Adult Health) study. *J Am Coll Cardiol.* 2009;53(10):860–869.

54. Shah AS, ghormli LEl, Bacha F, et al. Arterial stiffness: relationship to diabetes treatment and glycemic control in adolescents with type 2 diabetes (t2d) in the today clinical trial. In: *ADA 76th Scientific Sessions Annual Meeting, New Orleans, LA.;* 2016.

CHAPTER 8

Diabetic Retinopathy in Youth-Onset Type 2 Diabetes Mellitus

ERIN RICHARDSON, MD • RYAN FARRELL, MD

INTRODUCTION

With the high prevalence of obesity in children and adolescents, there has been an increase in the incidence of youth-onset type 2 diabetes mellitus (T2DM).[1,2] One of the primary concerns with the increase in T2DM diagnosed at a young age is complications since these youth will have many years of hyperglycemia exposure. Diabetic retinopathy (DR) is a microvascular complication of diabetes and is currently the leading cause of blindness in working-age adults in the United States.[3] Although vision-threatening retinopathy has historically been seen in adults, changes may happen earlier in youth-onset T2DM.

The risk of vision loss in young adulthood has major societal implications. Vision loss not only adversely affects an individual's ability to work but also to perform daily activities of living.[4] In addition, vision loss has more of an impact on quality of life than other risk factors in patients with diabetes.[5] Thus, prevention or early detection is critical.

This chapter will address what is known about DR in adolescents with T2DM. As there remains limited information for this population, insight from studies in adolescents with type 1 diabetes mellitus (T1DM) or adults with T2DM will also be included. A better understanding of the pathogenesis of youth-onset T2DM will guide screening recommendations and identify potential therapeutic targets for improved management in the future.

PATHOGENESIS AND NATURAL COURSE

Diabetic retinopathy refers to the changes in the retinal neurovascular unit in patients with diabetes.[6] It is classified based on changes to the microvasculature as nonproliferative (mild, moderate, or severe), and proliferative.[7,8] In addition, diabetic macular edema may present at any time.[7,8] Mild, only microaneurysms present, and moderate nonproliferative retinopathy

do not threaten vision and regression of lesions has been observed.[8] The neovascularization that characterizes proliferative diabetic retinopathy comprises fragile vessels at risk of rupturing.[8] This stage is vision threatening.[8] Macular edema, with increased exudate and swelling from impaired retinal microvascular function, is also vision threatening.[8]

Retinal neurons, glia, and vasculature may be affected by chronic hyperglycemia.[6] Although changes to the neurovascular unit likely start earlier, microaneurysms from pericyte (retinal capillary smooth muscle cell) loss are usually the first clinical sign of DR (Table 8.1).[6,9,10] Then, damaged capillaries leak lipoproteins that eventually lead to retinal edema and vascular compromise.[6,11] With progression, perfusion is impaired and retinal ischemia develops.[9] Changes from microvascular damage are seen on exam (Fig. 8.1).[6,9] For example, cotton-wool spots result from retinal ischemic changes and venous beading from venule dilatation.[6] The damaged vessels have increased permeability that can lead to retinal thickening and/or exudates.[9] The retina has high metabolic demands, so ischemia from capillary nonperfusion in more severe DR stimulates neovascularization, the hallmark of proliferative retinopathy.[7,12] This secondary proliferation of new vessels into the vitreous are prone to rupture and result in hemorrhage followed by the formation of fibrous bands, which ultimately cause traction and retinal detachment.[9]

There are four classes of retinal cells: vascular cells (pericytes, endothelial cells), macroglial cells (Muller cells, astrocytes), microglial cells, and neural cells (photoreceptors, bipolar cells, amacrine cells, ganglion cells) and all are affected by diabetes (Fig. 8.2).[13] Astroglia and Muller cells are retinal glial cells that work closely with retinal neurons to maintain their health and support them metabolically.[12] These macroglial cells lose their ability to maintain the blood-retinal barrier and increase production of cytokines including vascular endothelial growth factor

Pediatric Type II Diabetes. https://doi.org/10.1016/B978-0-323-55138-0.00008-5

TABLE 8.1
Management Options for Diabetic Retinopathy[a]

Level of DR	EVALUATION			TREATMENT			Follow-up Interval (Months; Approx)
	Fundus Photo	OCT Exam	Fluorescein Angiography	Intravitreal anti-VEGF	Focal Photocoagulation	Scatter Photocoagulation	
None	No	No	No	No	No	No	12
MILD NPDR: MICROANEURYSMS ONLY; RISK OF PDR 5% (1 YEAR) AND 14% (3 YEAR)							
–ME	Occasional	Yes	Occasional	No	No	No	12
+ME	Occasional	Yes	Occasional	Yes	Yes or no along with anti-VEGF	No	1–3
MODERATE NPDR: MICROANEURYSMS AND OTHER MICROVASCULAR LESIONS, BUT NOT SEVERE NPDR; RISK OF PDR 12%–26% (1 YEAR) AND 30%–48% (3 YEAR)							
–ME	Occasional	Yes	Occasional	No	No	No	6–12
+ME	Occasional	Yes	Occasional	Yes	Yes or no along with anti-VEGF	No	1–3
SEVERE NPDR: >20 HEMORRHAGES IN FOUR QUADRANTS OR VENOUS BEADING IN TWO QUADRANTS OR MICROVASCULAR LESIONS IN ONE OR MORE QUADRANTS, BUT NO PDR; RISK OF PDR 52% (1 YEAR) AND 71% (3 YEAR)							
–ME	Occasional	Yes	Occasional	No	No	Consider	2–3
+ME	Occasional	Yes	Likely	Yes	Yes or no along with anti-VEGF	Consider	1–3
VERY SEVERE NPDR: MULTIPLE CRITERIA MET FOR SEVERE NPDR							
–ME	Occasional	Yes	Likely	No	No	Consider	2–3
+ME	Occasional	Yes	Likely	Yes	Yes or no along with anti-VEGF	Consider	1–3
EARLY PDR: NEW BLOOD VESSEL FORMATION, PRERETINAL OR VITREOUS HEMORRHAGE; DOES NOT MEET CRITERIA FOR HIGH RISK PDR							
–ME	Occasional	Yes	Likely	No	No	Likely	2–3
+ME	Occasional	Yes	Likely	Yes	Yes or no along with anti-VEGF	Likely	1–3
HIGH RISK PDR: MILD NEOVASCULARIZATION OF OPTIC DISC+VITREOUS HEMORRHAGE, MODERATE TO SEVERE NEOVASCULARIZATION ± VITREOUS HEMORRHAGE, MODERATE NEOVASCULARIZATION ELSEWHERE WITH VITREOUS HEMORRHAGE							
–ME	Occasional	Yes	Likely	No	No	Yes	2–3
+ME	Occasional	Yes	Likely	Yes	Yes or no along with anti-VEGF	Yes	1–3
Severe PDR	Photos/OCT/fluorescein angiogram/ultrasound as indicated			Panretinal photocoagulation, focal laser, vitrectomy with endolaser, and anti-VEGF as indicated			

DR, diabetic retinopathy; *OCT*, optical coherence tomography; *VEGF*, vascular endothelial growth factor; *NPDR*, nonproliferative diabetic retinopathy; *PDR*, proliferative diabetic retinopathy; *–ME*, macular edema absent; *+ME*, macular edema present.
[a]Precise management guidelines have not yet been established at the time of this writing. This table summarizes current recommendations of Donald J D'Amico, MD and Szilard Kiss, MD and includes modifications from earlier recommendations from: Aiello LM. Perspectives on diabetic retinopathy. Am J Ophthalmol 2003; 136:122.

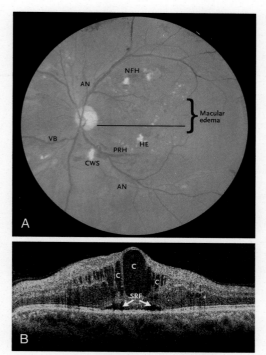

FIG. 8.1 Clinical findings in DR (Ref. 6). Panel A is a photograph of the fundus and B is an image from optical coherence tomography demonstrating clinically significant macular edema (Ref. 6). *AN*, arteriolar narrowing; *NFH*, nerve-fiber hemorrhage; *HE*, hard exudates; *CWS*, cotton-wool spots; *VB*, venous beading; *PRH*, preretinal hemorrhage; *C*, cyst; *SRF*, subretinal fluid (Ref. 6).

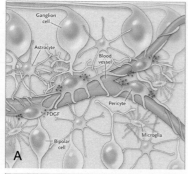

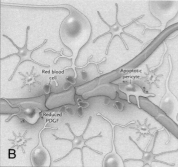

FIG. 8.2 Changes to the neovascular unit from diabetes (Ref. 6). Panel A depicts the normal cellular architecture and interactions of the neurovascular retina. Panel B demonstrates changes to the neovascular unit from diabetes. Loss of platelet-derived growth factor (PDGF) secretion and pericyte apoptosis lead to capillary permeability and degeneration, which in turn alters retinal perfusion (Ref. 6).

(VEGF) in diabetes.[13] By affecting protein expression at the tight junctions of the blood-retinal barrier, VEGF increases vascular permeability and may lead to macular edema.[13] Microglia are activated in diabetes and produce proinflammatory cytokines, which likely contribute to capillary degeneration and increased vascular permeability.[13]

The underlying pathology is complex (Fig. 8.3).[7] It has been suggested that retinal neural cell apoptosis precedes vascular apoptosis similar to what has been observed in rats with diabetes.[14] Glutamate excitotoxicity is hypothesized to be involved with neurodegeneration via excitotoxic cell death.[14] Glutamate accumulates in the extracellular space of retinal cells because of both impaired uptake and decreased enzymatic degradation in the setting of diabetes.[14] To compensate, glutamate receptors may be downregulated.[14] The altered neurotransmission may not only lead to apoptosis but may also impair visual signal processing.[14]

Previous research has shown inclusion of multifocal electroretinogram (mfERG) implicit times in multivariate models helps to predict specific areas of DR in the future.[15] The authors reported that this was likely due to impaired retinal bipolar cell function at the time retinopathy develops or possibly prior to development of retinopathy.[15] As retinal neuropathy may help predict future microvascular changes, retinal neural and vascular health of adolescents with T2DM was assessed.[16] Adolescents with T2DM had significantly delayed mfERG implicit times, retinal thinning, and dilation of retinal venules when compared to control adolescents without diabetes.[16] Potentially, some of these changes are a result of comorbidities such as obesity, hypertension, and hyperlipidemia frequently present in patients with type 2 diabetes mellitus.[16]

Based on experimental models, impaired trophic signaling pathways is another hypothesis for vascular and neural cell apoptosis.[14] Changes in supportive

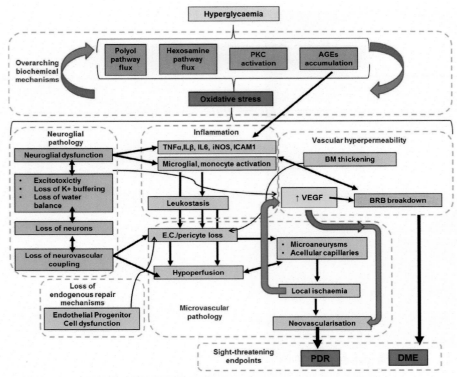

FIG. 8.3 Proposed pathogenic cascades in diabetic retinopathy (Ref. 7).

factors such as growth factors and/or expression of their receptors may increase the risk of cell apoptosis following stressful situations.[14] There is decreased production of the neuroprotective factors such as somatostatin and pigment epithelial-derived factor (PEDF) in patients with diabetes.[12] Somatostatin is neuroprotective and antiangiogenic, so it protects against proliferative diabetic retinopathy and macular edema.[17] It is downregulated in early stages of DR.[17]

Another potential cause of apoptosis is from hyperglycemia-induced oxidative stress.[14] Multiple processes causing tissue damage result from increased mitochondrial production of superoxide.[18] The mitochondrial uncoupling protein 2 helps to control reactive oxygen species in the mitochondria.[19] It has been shown that the risk of proliferative diabetic retinopathy is increased with uncoupling protein 2 gene polymorphisms in patients with diabetes.[20] There is also increased oxidative stress due to reduced bioavailable nitric oxide from increased arginase activity.[21] Advanced glycation end products from diabetes mellitus lead to production of reactive oxygen species that decreases vascular permeability.[12] Abnormal vascular permeability may result

in macular edema.[12] By leading to inflammation, reactive oxygen species also indirectly contribute to tissue destruction.[22]

In later stages of retinopathy, VEGF and erythropoietin (EPO) are produced from low oxygen levels in the retina.[12] These factors stimulate development of fragile new vessels on the retinal surface.[12] VEGF is a major contributor to the pathogenesis of diabetic retinopathy.[12]

Inflammation plays a critical role in the pathology of DR.[22] Compromised vessels and tight junctions from cytokines as well as leukostasis from chemokine recruitment contribute to diabetic retinopathy pathogenesis.[22]

EPIDEMIOLOGY

As the incidence of youth-onset T2DM increases, more studies are being conducted to understand DR timing and risk factors in this population. Early studies suggested DR did not develop until adulthood. Pima Indians of the Gila River Indian Community have the highest incidence of noninsulin-dependent diabetes mellitus (NIDDM) in the world.[23] A study completed between October 1983 and November 1987 to assess the incidence of proliferative retinopathy in subjects (at least 50% Pima, Papago, or a mixture of the tribes) 9 years of age and older with NIDDM in this community found all subjects diagnosed with proliferative retinopathy were at least 35 years old.[24] As diabetes duration increased, the incidence of proliferative retinopathy increased until reaching a peak at 15–20 years from diagnosis.[24] The cumulative incidence of proliferative retinopathy was 14.1% after 20 years of diabetes.[24] There was a greater incidence in younger subjects with diabetes for a similar length of time.[24] A substantial number of those with youth-onset NIDDM will have microvascular complications as young adults.[25] All subjects with proliferative retinopathy developed nonproliferative retinopathy first.[24]

In a large study of subjects with T1DM, the Diabetes Control and Complications Trial (DCCT) demonstrated that intensive diabetes treatment reduces complication risk.[26] The DCCT randomized patients with T1DM to intensive treatment (at least four blood glucose checks and three insulin injections daily as well as frequent dose adjustments based on blood glucose monitoring) or conventional treatment (daily urine or blood glucose check and one to two insulin injections as per standard of care in the 1980s).[26] The risk for microvascular complications was significantly reduced with improved glycemic control from intensive treatment.[26] For the adolescent population, the odds ratio for progression through at least three steps in the Early Treatment of Diabetic Retinopathy Study retinopathy level was decreased by 66% when comparing those in the intensive treatment group to those in the conventional treatment group.[27] The Epidemiology of Diabetes Interventions and Complications (EDIC) study followed subjects after the DCCT study ended.[28] Although subjects from the two treatment arms had similar hemoglobin A1c levels after 4 years, those from the intensive treatment group continued to have a lower risk of microvascular complications.[27] For the adolescent population, there was 74% less retinopathy progression in those from the intensive treatment group than in those from the conventional treatment group during the first 4 years of EDIC.[27] Unfortunately, this metabolic memory benefit did not persist after 10 years in the adolescent group.[29]

A study in Australia comparing patients with T2DM diagnosed between 15 and 30 years of age to patients with T1DM diagnosed between 15 and 30 years of age found no statistically significant difference in retinopathy prevalence.[30] For this study, direct fundoscopy under mydriasis or retinal photography records from the Royal Prince Alfred Hospital Diabetes Database were used to assess for DR.[30] The average diabetes duration was 11.6 years for those with T2DM and 14.7 years for those with T1DM.[30]

Globally, other studies have shown an increased prevalence in adolescents with T2DM and an increased risk of complications from diabetes in youth with T2DM when compared to youth with T1DM and without diabetes.[31] A study from India assessing subjects diagnosed with diabetes between 10 and 25 years of age found the incidence of DR to be 78/1000 person years in those with T2DM and 77.4/1000 person years in those with T1DM.[32] In this study, glutamic acid decarboxylase antibodies were positive in 5.6% of subjects with T2DM; this is important because some studies classify diabetes in an adolescent with at least one diabetes-related autoantibody, including glutamic acid decarboxylase, as T1DM.[32] After adjusting for relevant covariates, the study found that youth with T2DM had a 2.11 times higher risk of developing a complication of diabetes, not retinopathy specifically.[32] This finding implies that T2DM may be more aggressive than T1DM.[32]

The SEARCH study assessed youth (diagnosed before 20 years of age) with diabetes mellitus for more than 5 years (mean 6.8 years) using nonmydriatic retinal photography for DR.[33] The prevalence of DR was 42% for adolescents with T2DM compared to 17% for adolescents with T1DM.[33] The mean time since diabetes diagnosis was 7.2 years for those with T2DM and 6.8 years for those with T1DM.[33] Subjects with DR had significantly higher hemoglobin A1c and low-density lipoprotein (LDL) levels.[33] The prevalence of DR was lower in non-Hispanic white youth than youth of other race/ethnicities.[33] The majority of subjects with T2DM were of a race/ethnicity other than non-Hispanic white.[33]

The more recent observations from SEARCH from over 13 years report on 272 participants with T2DM with an average age of 22.1 years and diabetes duration of 7.9 years.[34] Although the average diabetes duration was the same for both T1DM and T2DM groups, the participants with T2DM were older at diagnosis and at the outcome visit.[34] Only 26.5% of those with T2DM were non-Hispanic white.[34] A nonmydriatic camera was used for fundus images.[34] The DR prevalence estimated at 21 years of age was 9.1% for those with T2DM and 5.6% for those with T1DM.[34] This difference was statistically significant.[34] Separating participants with T2DM by race/ethnicity revealed that the DR prevalence estimated at 21 years of age was much lower for non-Hispanic whites at 3.7% compared to all other races/ethnicities at 11.2%.[34] Those with T2DM had significantly higher odds (odds ratio 2.24) of developing DR compared to those with T1DM after controlling for established risk factors.[34] The retinopathy odds ratio was attenuated when the logistic regression model included mean arterial pressure suggesting that high blood pressure may affect the prevalence difference between those with T2DM versus T1DM.[34]

The Treatment Options for type 2 Diabetes in Adolescents and Youth (TODAY) study evaluated adolescents at an average age of 18.1 ±2.5 years with T2DM for 2–8 years (mean 4.9 ± 1.5 years) for retinopathy.[35] Eye exams with retinal photographs were completed the final year of the trial that had randomized subjects to one of three treatment groups: metformin, metformin and rosiglitazone, or metformin and intensive lifestyle intervention.[35] They found 13.7% of the participants had background retinopathy.[35] Severe nonproliferative and proliferative retinopathy were not found.[35] Risk factors included higher hemoglobin A1c levels, longer diabetes duration, and older age.[35] The prevalence of retinopathy was lower in the most obese subjects.[35]

Although advancements in treatment have resulted in improvements since the Wisconsin Epidemiologic Study of Diabetic Retinopathy (WESDR) started, there is still work to do.[36] In the early 1980s, WESDR started assessing subjects diagnosed with diabetes prior to age 30 years and taking insulin.[36] The study found a 17% prevalence of diabetic retinopathy in those with diabetes for fewer than 5 years and a 97.5% prevalence in those with diabetes for at least 15 years.[36] The estimated prevalence of DR in adults 40 years and older with diabetes in the United States in 2005–08 was 28.5%.[37] The prevalence was highest in non-Hispanic black subjects with diabetes at 38.8%.[37]

The increasing incidence of T2DM in youth is concerning.[2] A study from Japan found 135 of 1065 patients (12.7%) with early onset NIDDM (diagnosed before age 30 years) developed proliferative retinopathy before 35 years of age.[38] Proliferative retinopathy was present before the initial visit in 67% of these patients.[38] A study in Australia found that the odds ratio for retinopathy of 1.9 was greater in patients with T2DM diagnosed before 45 years of age than in those diagnosed later in life.[39] A recent study estimating morbidity and mortality reported that adolescents and young adults with T2DM may have severe complications by their 40s and may lose approximately 15 years of remaining life expectancy.[40]

DIAGNOSIS AND SCREENING FOR DIABETIC RETINOPATHY

The recommendation for DR screening in youth diagnosed with T2DM differs from that of youth diagnosed with T1DM, as comorbidities may already be present at diagnosis of T2DM given the often insidious onset of disease.[41] The American Diabetes Association, International Society for Pediatric and Adolescent Diabetes, American Academy of Pediatrics, and American Academy of Ophthalmology recommend all youth should be screened by an ophthalmologist or trained experienced observer with a dilated pupil exam for DR when initially diagnosed with T2DM and then at least annually.[8,9,41–44] Eye care professionals may recommend more or less frequent exams in certain situations.[41,42]

With time, research may better identify screening modalities and risk factors to suggest a more targeted screening schedule. For example, a recent study from the DCCT/EDIC Study Group recommended personalizing the frequency of retinopathy screening for patients with T1DM based on their current retinopathy state and glycemic control (hemoglobin A1c).[45]

Despite recommendations, a recent large retrospective study of insured youth with T2DM found that only 42.2% had undergone an eye exam in the 6 years following their diagnosis of T2DM.[46] Youth from a lower socioeconomic status and ethnic minorities were less likely to have the recommended eye exams.[46] This is concerning considering early detection is important for future outcomes. Thus, approaches to make screening more accessible may be beneficial. Some suggest that screening for diabetic retinopathy with a nonmydriatic fundus camera in the outpatient endocrinology clinic may be a more convenient opportunity to improve compliance with screening recommendations.[47]

CLINICAL PRESENTATION

Unfortunately, the clinical presentation of diabetic retinopathy in its early stages is insidious and without obvious symptomatology, which underscores the value of early screening, treatment, and prevention. In contrast to adults, the onset of retinopathy in children with T2D seems to be early and rapidly progressive. Currently, only later stages of diabetic retinopathy and clinically significant macular edema necessitate ophthalmologic interventions, but early identification of nonproliferative diabetic retinopathy allows more regular screening for progression and also allows more diverse options for risk factor management. Thus, it is critical to screen early in the disease course (at diagnosis). Those patients who fail to receive appropriate screening present instead with visual symptoms.

When symptoms are present, they indicate more advanced proliferative disease and/or macular edema. Patients that develop vitreous bleeding may complain of a sense of a falling curtain. Some individuals may have a sense of floaters, which may develop after vitreous bleeds. Often times, blood can be slowly reabsorbed, with subsequent spontaneous improvement in visual disturbances over months. Changes in visual acuity over time that fail to correct with refraction may suggest the development of macular edema.

OPHTHALMOLOPIC FEATURES

There are several classic features of diabetic retinopathy, of which the presence and quantity assist in the classification of the different severities of diabetic retinopathy. DR can be classified as either proliferative or nonproliferative:

Nonproliferative diabetic retinopathy (NPDR) generally is absent of neovascularization but has other defining features. Classification of severity is critical, as the staging of nonproliferative diabetic retinopathy may dictate the risk for development of proliferative diabetic retinopathy as well as the frequency of suggested follow-up. NPDR may be classified into different severities: mild, moderate, and severe. In mild nonproliferative diabetic retinopathy, typically only microaneurysms (at least one) are present. Development of cotton wool spots, hemorrhage/microaneurysm, or microvascular abnormalities signify moderate NPDR. Severe NPDR is defined by either hemorrhage/microaneurysm in all four quadrants, venous beading in at least two quadrants, or intraretinal microvascular abnormalities in at least one quadrant.

Proliferative diabetic retinopathy (PDR) is classified as either early, high-risk, or severe. Early PDR demonstrates new blood vessel formation or neovascularization but not significant enough to meet criteria for high-risk PDR. High-risk PDR shows at least 1/3 to 1/2 of the disk area with neovascularization, and vitreous or preretinal hemorrhage may also be present. When the posterior fundus is obscured by preretinal or vitreous hemorrhage, this constitutes severe PDR.

Any stage of diabetic retinopathy (either proliferative or nonproliferative) can be associated with clinically significant macular edema (CSME). This is defined as thickening of the retina <500 μm from the center of the macula, presence of hard exudates, or a zone of retinal thickening at least 1 disc area in size located less than 1 disc diameter from the macular center.

MANAGEMENT
Prevention/Control of Risk Factors

Control of glycemia: It has been well established because of the DCCT that tighter glycemic control impacts progression rates of retinopathy in patients with T1DM.[26] Analogous observations have been seen for type 2 diabetes as part of the United Kingdom Prospective Diabetes Study (UKPDS), which demonstrated the lower risk of microvascular complications with an A1c of 7%.[48] Adults with T2D tend to have lower risks for retinopathy, especially those individuals not requiring insulin therapy and who are over the age of 30.[49] However, it is clear that youth with T2D have a more aggressive condition that in turn is accompanied by a higher risk of retinopathy.[50] Progression rates in individuals with T2D diagnosed in childhood are being investigated longitudinally currently in the TODAY2 study (a continuation of the TODAY study).

Control of hypertension: Several studies have examined the potential impact of blood pressure management on progression or development of diabetic retinopathy. Control of systemic blood pressure has been previously demonstrated to be beneficial in adults with T2D, based on results from the United Kingdom Prospective Diabetes Study.[51] Over 1000 patients with type 2 diabetes were randomized to receive tight blood pressure control versus less tight control. Those individuals who had tighter blood pressure control demonstrated a 34% reduction in progression of diabetic retinopathy and a 47% reduction in the risk of deterioration in visual acuity. A Cochrane review also confirmed that lowering blood pressure may have benefits in preventing DR at four–5 years, but evidence was modest and there was insufficient evidence to recommend BP management to slow progression of retinopathy.[52] The ACCORD study also evaluated the effect of BP control on DR. Patients without DR at baseline did not have improved prevention of DR with BP control with goal systolic blood pressure (SBP) of <120. In subjects with DR at baseline, BP control also failed to show benefit in minimizing progression of DR, while tight glycemic control (A1c <6%) did show reduction in DR progression, particularly in mild NPDR.[53]

Control of Hyperlipidemia: The effects of lipid control on DR progression are poorly established, but there are suggestions in the literature that there may be at least some modest beneficial effect. Medications that have looked at both triglycerides as well as LDL have been studied to some degree. Fenofibrate, often used to treat hypertriglyceridemia, may also have some additional effects to reduce inflammation and angiogenesis as well.[54] A large study (FIELD study) of 1012 patients with T2D demonstrated that individuals treated with fenofibrate had lower rates of requiring photocoagulation and lower rates of progression compared to those without fenofibrate.[55] It is unclear if this effect was mediated by the lowering of triglycerides, the antiinflammatory and antiangiogenic properties, or both.

A small and short trial followed 50 subjects with DM (both type 1 and type 2) and hypercholesterolemia for 6 months.[56] Compared to placebo, those individuals treated with simvastatin showed less deterioration in visual acuity. Subjects in the placebo group also showed deterioration in findings on angiography compared to those treated with a statin. Individuals with T2D benefit from improved lipid control for many reasons, but it appears that there may be at least some modest effect on the development of DR.

Ophthalmologic Treatments

Laser Photocoagulation: The current indications for laser photocoagulation in diabetic retinopathy include retinal neovascularization (PDR) and clinically significant (Fig. 8.4) macular edema. Presently, laser photocoagulation continues to be among the most common therapies for diabetic retinopathy. Laser photocoagulation may consist of pan-retinal photocoagulation in the setting of proliferative retinopathy, or it may consist of macular or focal photocoagulation in the setting of diabetic macular edema. Although photocoagulation is primarily used in proliferative diabetic retinopathy, under some circumstances (particularly in individuals with T2D), it may be prudent to treat more severe cases of NPDR that are at higher risk for rapid progression to PDR.[57] Individual circumstances, including current glycemic control, risk of poor follow-up, and the disease status of the fellow eye, may influence the decision to proceed with panretinal photocoagulation prior to development of PDR.

Panretinal photocoagulation has been studied extensively. Compared to untreated eyes, eyes treated with panretinal photocoagulation had 50% reduction in severe vision loss by 6 years posttreatment.[58] Similar rates of neovascular regression have also been seen after treatment, with higher rates of regression being noted in individuals with better glycemic control (Fig. 8.4).

The evidence to support the use of laser photocoagulation of the treatment of diabetic retinopathy stems from two pivotal clinical trials: The Diabetic Retinopathy Study (DRS) and the Early Treatment Diabetic Retinopathy Study (ETDRS). The DRS enrolled over 1700 patients with proliferative diabetic retinopathy. Over the course of 5 years, those individuals treated with pan retinal photocoagulation had a 50% reduction in risk of severe visual loss.[58] The ETDRS enrolled an additional 3700 patients. These individuals had less severe

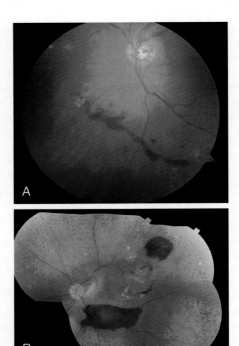

FIG. 8.4 **(A)** Image of left eye showing neovascularization of the disc (NVD) and preretinal hemorrhage from preretinal neovascularization. **(B)** Montage of left eye of another patient who had panretinal photocoagulation and with preretinal hemorrhage and fibrovascular membranes on the macula. (**(A)** Courtesy of Cyrie Fry, CRA, OCT-C. **(B)** Courtesy of James Gilman, CRA, FOPS. 2017 Mary Elizabeth Hartnett. All Rights Reserved.[59])

diabetic retinopathy (NPDR or early proliferative) compared to subjects enrolled in the DRS. Although panretinal photocoagulation did lower risk in subjects with milder NPDR, controls had low progression rates and the conclusions from this study were to defer treatment in mild-to-moderate NPDR.[60] The use of focal photocoagulation in ETDRS showed beneficial impacts in subjects with CSME, with moderate vision loss being reduced by half.[61] When focal photocoagulation is performed, it can be targeted to specific lesions or performed nonspecifically in areas of edema. Care must be made to have at least 500 μm of space between the laser and the fovea, as accidental coagulation of the fovea may decrease visual acuity. However, treatment is quick and can be performed with topical anesthesia. Edema may take several weeks or longer to improve.

Although photocoagulation is highly effective in more severe forms of DR, adverse effects are not infrequent. Upwards of 25% of individuals will have light dark-adaptation difficulties.[62] Some will still report decreases in visual acuity and peripheral visual loss. Less frequently, changes in color vision and worsening of macular edema have also been reported. Nevertheless, panretinal photocoagulation remains the gold standard of treatment for proliferative diabetic retinopathy.

Corticosteroids: Intravitreal triamcinolone has been used dating back to the 1980s for management of CSME; its effects include reduction in VEGF levels and inhibition of ICAM-1 production.[63] However, use of triamcinolone is associated with high risks of complications, including cataract formation (over half of patients require cataract surgery),[64] ocular hypertension (requiring medication in over a quarter of patients),[65] and endophthalmitis, specifically with *strep viridans* (3 times higher rate compared to photocoagulation).[66] In addition to the higher rates of adverse effects, DRCR.net studies have not shown benefit of steroids at 3 years posttreatment compared to photocoagulation in CSME.[67] It is unclear if steroids may play a role as adjunct therapy when combined with photocoagulation. Similarly, corticosteroid treatment has been investigated in the treatment of PDR. Although triamcinolone has positive effects on neovascularization, its aforementioned side effects continue to preclude its use given the alternative options currently available.

Anti-VEGF: The use of antivascular endothelial growth factor treatments has stemmed from the known pathophysiologic role of VEGF, which was first noted in the 1990s. As of 2015, four anti-VEGF agents have been studied in the treatment of diabetic retinopathy.[54] Presently, anti-VEGF treatment has become first-line therapy for clinically significant macular edema. Multiple large, multi-center clinical trials have demonstrated the effectiveness of anti-VEGF intravitreal injections. Use of anti-VEGF medications has been associated with long-term improvements in visual acuity and has also been associated with decreased central retinal subfield thickness on optical coherence tomography (OCT), even when compared to laser photocoagulation. Four different anti-VEG treatments have been studied in diabetic retinopathy:

1. Bevacizumab: Bevacizumab is a monoclonal antibody that nonselectively blocks VEGF isoforms. It has been used in various different malignancies including colon cancer and nonsmall cell lung cancer. It can also be used to treat diabetic macular edema (DME), but this is an off-label use. It is sometimes used as adjunctive therapy in other circumstances (see below). Adverse reactions associated with the use of bevacizumab include hypertension, mucosal bleeding, proteinuria, neutropenia, gastrointestinal operations, and possible thromboembolic events.

2. Ranibizumab: This medication is also a monoclonal antibody that binds all VEGF subtypes. It is an FDA approved treatment of DME, although studies have shown that it may also lower rates of retinopathy deterioration and may actually improve retinopathy.[68] It is also associated with lower rates of proliferative diabetic retinopathy and may have a role in its prevention or management.

3. Aflibercept: This medication is FDA approved for the treatment of diabetic macular edema and diabetic retinopathy. It is a recombinant fusion protein made of the binding portion of VEGF receptors, which are then fused to an Fc portion of IgG. Studies using aflibercept in the treatment of DME have shown that in patients with lower visual acuity, it may be a more beneficial treatment than the other two previously mentioned anti-VEGF treatments.[69]

4. Pegaptanib: This medication is a selective inhibitor to VEGF-A165, which is the major isoform found in the eye. A 2009 study by Gonzalez and colleagues demonstrated 100% complete regression of neovascularization in patients with proliferative diabetic retinopathy, compared to only 25% of eyes treated with panretinal photocoagulation.[70] This regression has been seen in multiple studies, but presently pegaptanib is not FDA approved for treatment of DME or diabetic retinopathy.

The DRCR.net protocol T study, published in 2015, compared the effectiveness of aflibercept, ranibizumab, and bevacizumab in the treatment of clinically significant macular edema. Serious adverse event rates were similar among the three medications, but bevacizumab was inferior to both aflibercept and ranibizumab in measured outcomes. Results after 2 years of treatment demonstrated superiority of aflibercept over ranibizumab, particularly in patients that have worse baseline visual acuity. Aflibercept was also associated with reduced central subfield thickness on OCT compared to bevacizumab and ranibizumab.[69]

In some circumstances, anti-VEGF therapies may also serve as adjunct treatment in cases of proliferative diabetic retinopathy. For example, intravitreous ranibizumab demonstrated noninferiority to panretinal photocoagulation in 394 eyes with PDR, as measured by change in mean visual acuity.[71] In another study, a single injection of bevacizumab (compared to a sham injection) was given at the time of panretinal photocoagulation treatment.[72] Those subjects treated with adjunct bevacizumab showed complete regression of PDR at 6 weeks (compared to 25% in sham).

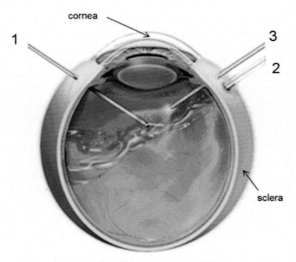

FIG. 8.5 Typical three-port pars plana vitrectomy procedure: the aspiration pipe (the so-called "vitrector") (1) allows slow removal of the natural vitreous; the infusion pipe (2) is used to replace the vitreous with an appropriate substitute; the light pipe (3) is useful to the surgeon for exploring the vitreous cavity and for examining the retina.[77]

Unfortunately, this regression was temporary and by 16 weeks rates of regression between the two groups were similar. Bevacizumab has also been used as a pretreatment prior to vitrectomy. Subjects treated with bevacizumab had lower rates of recurrent vitreous cavity hemorrhage.[73]

Generally, adverse reactions associated with VEGF inhibitors are relatively infrequent, with the most common being elevations in intraocular pressure, occurring in up to 12% of patients.[69] Additional side defects including endophthalmitis occur in under 1% of subjects. Initial concerns regarding higher stroke risk or mortality effects have not been substantiated.[74,75] Risk of bleeding is generally low, including in individuals that are taking antiplatelet or anticoagulant medications such as aspirin (Fig. 8.5).[76]

Surgical Intervention

Indications for vitrectomy (Fig. 8.5) arise from complications of PDR and include vitreous hemorrhage, traction retinal detachment that involves the fovea, traction/rhegmatogenous retinal detachment, rubeosis (neovascularization of the iris), which may preclude panretinal photocoagulation, and in neovascularization unresponsive to photocoagulation.[78] Ongoing vessel proliferation increases risk for visual loss from vitreous hemorrhage. In circumstances of vitreous hemorrhage that does not resolve, removal of the vitreous humor with accompanying photocoagulation may improve vision, depending on the extent of retinal disease. In situations of vitreal contraction, retinal detachments due to traction may occur. Particularly when involving the fovea, this can threaten vision. In individuals with isolated vitreous hemorrhage, vitrectomy improves vision in the majority of circumstances. This is also true in individuals with traction retinal detachment that involves the fovea. The Diabetic Retinopathy Vitrectomy Study (DRVS) was published in the late 1980s, and it demonstrated that early vitrectomy may provide better preservation of sight over several years, particularly in cases of advanced PDR.[79]

Vitrectomy has been studied in the management of CSME as well, particularly when it fails to respond to focal photocoagulation. A 2009 study by Kralinger showed improvement in visual acuity from 20/320 to 20/80 in cases of CSME treated with vitrectomy.[80] A smaller study by Stolba showed improvement in vitrectomy-treated eyes compared to observation alone. All eyes had grid laser photocoagulation performed at least 4 months earlier.[81] In circumstances of CSME with accompanying macular traction, vitrectomy may also be a therapeutic option, although visual outcomes have been inconsistent with inconsistent evidence. In general, vitrectomy may be a consideration in cases of CSME failing to respond to more conventional treatments such as VEGF inhibitors or laser therapy.

Complications of vitrectomy include cataract development (seen more frequently in older individuals), along with small risks of retinal detachment and endophthalmitis.

Follow-up

Frequency of follow-up ophthalmologic evaluation in patients with established diabetic retinopathy are dependent on staging and coexisting consultations. In individuals with no retinopathy, annual or biannual assessment may be sufficient. In individuals with mild or moderate NPDR without macular edema, risk continues to remain low for progression to PDR, and annual surveillance may be appropriate. However, in cases of more severe NPDR, risk of progression to PDR increases dramatically, and these individuals must be monitored quite closely. In addition, CSME can develop at any stage of DR and also warrants regular monitoring and intervention.

Future Studies and Emerging Therapies

Despite the success of photocoagulation and intravitreal medications, many individuals still have adverse reactions and/or lack of clinical improvement. There remains an ongoing need for additional therapies to potentially prevent progression of diabetic retinopathy.

Somatostatin is currently being investigated as part of a European phase II/III study in the treatment of NPDR. Somatostatin has neuroprotective effects and appears to be in lower levels in patients with PDR or DME. Previous small studies have demonstrated in severe NPDR or early PDR that somatostatin analogs minimized need for panretinal photocoagulation.[82,83] In addition, preliminary results from the EUROCONDOR study show that somatostatin and brimonidine arrested neurodegeneration progression compared to placebo, but brimonidine in particular was associated with frequent local adverse effects, which may limit its potential benefit.[84]

Sulodexide is an oral glycosaminoglycan that has demonstrated some beneficial effects on hard exudates in subjects with NPDR.[85] It is considered that GAG supplementation may minimize collagen deposition at the basement membrane, which affects vascular permeability. Additional oral supplements may also have effects and are being studied in more detail.

Angiopoietin 2 has been implicated in development of CSME due to its effects on angiogenesis and vascular permeability. AKB-9778 is a potential drug targeting the effects of angiopoietin 2 to attempt to reduce vascular permeability. Initial trials show a good safety profile with evidence of reduction in OCT thickness in patients with DME.[86]

Small interfering RNAs (siRNAs) are being investigated as well. These molecules can bind to specific genes and prevent expression. Bevasiranib is being investigated as an siRNA that inhibits expression of VEGF, and this treatment has shown reductions in OCT thickness in subjects with DME.[87]

Luminate is another novel molecule that leads a class of antiintegrin treatments. Integrins are cell adhesion and signaling receptors that have been implicated in retinal angiogenesis. It has been shown to be safe and resulted in visual improvement in 50% of subjects, lowering OCT thickness by 83%.[88] This may result in another target by which to prevent angiogenesis.

CONCLUSIONS

Diabetic retinopathy continues to affect older populations, and the identification of more youth, particularly minority youth, with DR at the time of diagnosis suggests that these children must be closely screened. These subjects, who also come from lower socioeconomic backgrounds, are highly susceptible to being

lost to follow-up, and failure to identify evolving PDR or CSME may result in missed opportunities to preserve vision. Although the mainstays of treatment continue to be prevention along with photocoagulation, the development of anti-VEGF therapies as mainstream treatment and the promising future of specific targeted therapies may allow for a large arsenal of medical options that allow for earlier intervention and are less invasive and increasingly effective.

REFERENCES

1. Ogden CL, Carroll MD, Kit BK, Flegal KM. Prevalence of childhood and adult obesity in the United States, 2011–2012. *JAMA*. 2014;311(8):806–814.
2. Mayer-Davis EJ, Lawrence JM, Dabelea D, et al. SEARCH for Diabetes in Youth Study. Incidence trends of type 1 and type 2 diabetes among youths, 2002–2012. *N Engl J Med*. 2017;376(15):1419–1429.
3. Centers for Disease Control and Prevention. *National Diabetes Fact Sheet: National Estimates and General Information on Diabetes and Prediabetes in the United States*. Atlanta, GA: U.S. Department of Health and Human Services, Centers for Disease Control and Prevention, 2011; 2011.
4. Lamoureux EL, Hassell JB, Keeffe JE. The impact of diabetic retinopathy on participation in daily living. *Arch Ophthalmol*. 2004;122:84–88.
5. Gubitosi-Klug RA, Sun W, Cleary PA, et al. DCCT/EDIC research group. Effects of prior intensive insulin therapy and risk factors on visual quality-of-life in the diabetes control and complications trial/epidemiology of diabetes interventions and complications (DCCT/EDIC) cohort. *JAMA Ophthalmol*. 2016;134(2):137–145.
6. Antonetti DA, Klein R, Gardner TW. Diabetic retinopathy. *N Engl J Med*. 2012;366:1227–1239.
7. Lechner J, O'Leary OE, Stitt AW. The pathology associated with diabetic retinopathy. *Vis Res*. 2017;139:7–14.
8. Donaghue KC, Wadwa RP, Dimeglio LA, et al. Microvascular and macrovascular complications in children and adolescents. *Pediatr Diabetes*. 2014;15(suppl 20):257–269.
9. AAO PPP Retina/Vitreous Panel. *Hoskins Center for Quality Eye Care*. Diabetic retinopathy PPP; 2016. updated 2016 https://www.aao.org/preferred-practice-pattern/diabetic-retinopathy-ppp-updated-2016.
10. Stitt AW, Gardiner TA, Archer DB. Histological and ultrastructural investigation of retinal microaneurysm development in diabetic patients. *Br J Ophthalmol*. 1995;79:362–367.
11. Crandall J, Shamoon H. Diabetes Mellitus. In: 25th ed. Goldman L, Schafer AI, eds. *Goldman-cecil Medicine*. Vol. 229. Philadelphia, PA: Elsevier Saunders; 2016:1527–1548. e3.
12. Ben-Skowronek I. Growth factors in the pathogenesis of retinal neurodegeneration in diabetes mellitus. *Curr Neuropharmacol*. 2016;14(8):792–804.

13. Gardner TW, Antonetti DA, Barber AJ, LaNoue KF, Levison SW. The Penn state retina research group. Diabetic retinopathy: more than meets the eye. *Surv Ophthalmol.* 2002;47(suppl 2):S253–S262.
14. Barber AJ, Gardner TW, Abcouwer SF. The significance of vascular and neural apoptosis to the pathology of diabetic retinopathy. *Invest Ophthalmol Vis Sci.* 2011;52(2):1156–1163.
15. Han Y, Schneck ME, Bearse Jr MA, et al. Formulation and evaluation of a predictive model to identify the sites of future diabetic retinopathy. *Invest Ophthalmol Vis Sci.* 2004;45(11):4106–4112.
16. Bronson-Castain KW, Bearse Jr MA, Neuville J, et al. Adolescents with type 2 diabetes: early indications of focal retinal neuropathy, retinal thinning and venular dilation. *Retina.* 2009;29(5):618–626.
17. Hernandez C, Garcia-Ramirez M, Corraliza L, et al. Topical administration of somatostatin prevents retinal degeneration in experimental diabetes. *Diabetes.* 2013;62(7):2569–2578.
18. Giacco F, Brownlee M. Oxidative stress and diabetic complications. *Circ Res.* 2010;107:1058–1070.
19. Pi J, Collins S. Reactive oxygen species and uncoupling protein 2 in pancreatic beta-cell function. *Diabetes Obes Metab.* 2010;12(suppl 2):141–148.
20. Crispim D, Fagundes NJ, dos Santos KG, et al. Polymorphisms of the UCP2 gene are associated with proliferative diabetic retinopathy in patients with diabetes mellitus. *Clin Endocrinol (Oxf).* 2010;72(5):612–619.
21. Patel C, Rojas M, Narayanan SP, et al. Arginase as a mediator of diabetic retinopathy. *Front Immunol.* 2013;4:173.
22. Roy S, Kern TS, Song B, Stuebe C. Mechanistic insights into pathological changes in the diabetic retina. *Am J Pathol.* 2017;187:9–19.
23. Knowler WC, Bennett PH, Hamman RF, Miller M. Diabetes incidence and prevalence in Pima Indians: a 19-fold greater incidence than in Rochester, Minnesota. *Am J Epidemiol.* 1978;108(6):497–505.
24. Nelson RG, Wolfe JA, Horton MB, Pettitt DJ, Bennett PH, Knowler WC. Proliferative retinopathy in NIDDM. Incidence and risk factors in Pima Indians. *Diabetes.* 1989;38:435–440.
25. Krakoff J, Lindsay RS, Looker HC, Nelson RG, Hanson RL, Knowler WC. Incidence of retinopathy and nephropathy in youth-onset compared with adult-onset type 2 diabetes. *Diabetes Care.* 2003;26(1):76–81.
26. DCCT Research Group. The effect of intensive treatment of diabetes on the development and progression of long-term complications in insulin-dependent diabetes mellitus. *N Engl J Med.* 1993;329:977–986.
27. White NH, Cleary PA, Dahms W, et al. (DCCT)/Epidemiology of diabetes interventions and complications (EDIC) research group. Beneficial effects of intensive therapy of diabetes during adolescence: outcomes after the conclusion of the diabetes control and complications trial (DCCT). *J Pediatr.* 2001;139(6):804–812.
28. DCCT-EDIC Research Group. Retinopathy and nephropathy in patients with type I diabetes four years after a trial of intensive therapy. *N Engl J Med.* 2000;342:381–389.
29. White NH, Sun W, Cleary PA, et al. DCCT-EDIC Research Group. Effect of prior intensive therapy in type 1 diabetes on 10-year progression of retinopathy in the DCCT/EDIC: comparison of adults and adolescents. *Diabetes.* 2010;59(5):1244–1253.
30. Constantino MI, Molyneaux L, Limacher-Gisler F, et al. Long-term complications and mortality in young-onset diabetes: type 2 diabetes is more hazardous and lethal than type I diabetes. *Diabetes Care.* 2013;36(12):3863–3869.
31. Dart AB, Martens PJ, Rigatto C, Brownell MD, Dean HJ, Sellers EA. Earlier onset of complications in youth with type 2 diabetes. *Diabetes Care.* 2014;37(2):436–443.
32. Amutha A, Anjana RM, Venkatesan U, et al. Incidence of complications in young-onset diabetes: comparing type 2 with type 1 (the young diab study). *Diabetes Res Clin Pract.* 2017;123:1–8.
33. Mayer-Davis EJ, Davis C, Saadine J, et al. The SEARCH for Diabetes in Youth Study Group. Diabetic retinopathy in the SEARCH for diabetes in youth cohort: a pilot study. *Diabetes Med.* 2012;29(9):1148–1152.
34. Dabelea D, Stafford JM, Mayer-Davis EJ, et al. SEARCH for Diabetes in Youth Research Group. Association of type 1 diabetes vs type 2 diabetes diagnosed during childhood and adolescence with complications during teenage years and young adulthood. *JAMA.* 2017;317(8):825–835.
35. TODAY Study Group. Retinopathy in youth with type 2 diabetes participating in the TODAY clinical trial. *Diabetes Care.* 2013;36(6):1772–1774.
36. Klein R, Klein BE, Moss SE, Davis MD, DeMets DL. The Wisconsin Epidemiologic Study of Diabetic Retinopathy. II. Prevalence and risk of diabetic retinopathy when age at diagnosis is less than 30 years. *Arch Opthalmol.* 1984;102(4):520–526.
37. Zhang X, Saaddine JB, Chou CF, et al. Prevalence of diabetic retinopathy in the United States, 2005-2008. *JAMA.* 2010;304(6):649–656.
38. Yokoyama H, Okudaira M, Otani T, et al. Existence of early-onset NIDDM Japanese demonstrating severe diabetic complications. *Diabetes Care.* 1997;20(5):844–847.
39. Wong J, Molyneaux L, Constantino M, Twigg SM, Yue DK. Timing is everything: age of onset influences long-term retinopathy risk in type 2 diabetes, independent of traditional risk factors. *Diabetes Care.* 2008;31(10):1985–1990.
40. Rhodes ET, Prosser LA, Hoerger TJ, Lieu T, Ludwig DS, Laffel LM. Estimated morbidity and mortality in adolescents and young adults diagnosed with type 2 diabetes mellitus. *Diabetes Med.* 2012;29(4):453–463.
41. American Diabetes Association. Children and adolescents. Sec. 12. In standards of medical care in Diabetes—2017. *Diabetes Care.* 2017;40(suppl 1):S105–S113.
42. Springer SC, Silverstein J, Copeland K, et al. Technical report: management of type 2 diabetes mellitus in children and adolescents. *Pediatrics.* 2013;131:e648–e664.

43. Zeitler P, Fu J, Tandon N, et al. Type 2 diabetes in the child and adolescent. *Pediatr Diabetes.* 2014;15(suppl 20): 26–46.

44. Geloneck MM, Forbes BJ, Shaffer J, Ying G, Binenbaum G. Ocular complications in children with diabetes mellitus. *Ophthalmology.* 2015;122:2457–2464.

45. DCCT-EDIC Research Group, Nathan DM, Bebu I, et al. Frequency of evidence-based screening for retinopathy in type 1 diabetes. *N Engl J Med.* 2017;376(16): 1507–1516.

46. Wang SY, Andrews CA, Gardner TW, Wood M, Singer K, Stein JD. Ophthalmic screening patterns among youths with diabetes enrolled in a large US managed care network. *JAMA Ophthalmol.* 2017;135(5):432–438.

47. Tapley JL, McGwin Jr G, Ashraf AP, et al. Feasibility and efficacy of diabetic retinopathy screening among youth with diabetes in a pediatric endocrinology clinic: a cross-sectional study. *Diabetol Metab Syndr.* 2015;7:56.

48. Stratton IM, Adler AI, Neil AW, et al. Association of Glycaemia with Macrovascular and Microvascular Complications of Type 2 Diabetes (UKPDS 35): Prospective Observational Study. https://www.ncbi.nlm.nih.gov/pmc/articles/PMC27454/pdf/405.pdf.

49. Klein R, Klein BE, Moss SE, Davis MD, DeMets DL. The Wisconsin epidemiologic study of diabetic retinopathy. III. Prevalence and risk of diabetic retinopathy when age at diagnosis is 30 or more years. *Arch Ophthalmol (Chicago, Ill 1960).* 1984;102(4):527–532. http://www.ncbi.nlm.nih.gov/pubmed/6367725.

50. Pinhas-Hamiel O, Zeitler P. Acute and chronic complications of type 2 diabetes mellitus in children and adolescents. *Lancet.* 2007;369(9575):1823–1831. https://doi.org/10.1016/S0140-6736(07)60821-6.

51. Tight blood pressure control and risk of macrovascular and microvascular complications in type 2 diabetes: UKPDS 38. UK Prospective Diabetes Study Group. *BMJ.* 1998;317(7160):703–713. https://doi.org/10.1136/BMJ.317.7160.703.

52. Do DV, Wang X, Vedula SS, et al. Blood pressure control for diabetic retinopathy. *Cochrane Database Syst Rev.* 2015;1:CD006127. https://doi.org/10.1002/14651858.CD006127.pub2.

53. Group TASG and AES. Effects of medical therapies on retinopathy progression in type 2 diabetes. *N Engl J Med.* 2010;363(3):233–244. https://doi.org/10.1056/NEJMoa1001288.

54. Vaziri K, Schwartz SG, Relhan N, Kishor KS, Flynn HW. New therapeutic approaches in diabetic retinopathy. *Rev Diabetes Stud.* 2015;12(1–2):196–210. https://doi.org/10.1900/RDS.

55. Keech AC, Mitchell P, Summanen PA, et al. Effect of fenofibrate on the need for laser treatment for diabetic retinopathy (FIELD study): a randomised controlled trial. *Lancet (London, England).* 2007;370(9600):1687–1697. https://doi.org/10.1016/S0140-6736(07)61607-9.

56. Sen K, Misra A, Kumar A, Pandey RM. Simvastatin retards progression of retinopathy in diabetic patients with hypercholesterolemia. *Diabetes Res Clin Pract.* 2002;56(1): 1–11. http://www.ncbi.nlm.nih.gov/pubmed/11879715.

57. Grading diabetic retinopathy from stereoscopic color fundus photographs–an extension of the modified Airlie House classification. ETDRS report number 10. Early treatment diabetic retinopathy study research group. *Ophthalmology.* 1991;98(suppl 5):786–806. http://www.ncbi.nlm.nih.gov/pubmed/2062513.

58. Photocoagulation treatment of proliferative diabetic retinopathy. Clinical application of diabetic retinopathy study (DRS) findings, DRS report number 8. The diabetic retinopathy study research group. *Ophthalmology.* 1981;88(7): 583–600. http://www.ncbi.nlm.nih.gov/pubmed/7196564.

59. Hartnett ME, Baehr W, Le YZ. Diabetic retinopathy, an overview. *Vis Res.* August 2017. https://doi.org/10.1016/j.visres.2017.07.006.

60. Early photocoagulation for diabetic retinopathy. ETDRS report number 9. Early treatment diabetic retinopathy study research group. *Ophthalmology.* 1991;98(suppl 5):766–785. http://www.ncbi.nlm.nih.gov/pubmed/2062512.

61. Photocoagulation for diabetic macular edema. Early treatment diabetic retinopathy study report number 1. Early treatment diabetic retinopathy study research group. *Arch Ophthalmol (Chicago, Ill 1960).* 1985;103(12):1796–1806. http://www.ncbi.nlm.nih.gov/pubmed/2866759.

62. Mohamed Q, Gillies MC, Wong TY. Management of diabetic retinopathy. *JAMA.* 2007;298(8):902. https://doi.org/10.1001/jama.298.8.902.

63. Matsuda S, Gomi F, Oshima Y, Tohyama M, Tano Y. Vascular endothelial growth factor reduced and connective tissue growth factor induced by triamcinolone in ARPE19 cells under oxidative stress. *Investig Opthalmology Vis Sci.* 2005;46(3):1062. https://doi.org/10.1167/iovs.04-0761.

64. Diabetic Retinopathy Clinical Research Network. A randomized trial comparing intravitreal triamcinolone acetonide and focal/grid photocoagulation for diabetic macular edema. *Ophthalmology.* 2008;115(9):1447–1459.e10. https://doi.org/10.1016/j.ophtha.2008.06.015.

65. Bakri SJ, Beer PM. The effect of intravitreal triamcinolone acetonide on intraocular pressure. *Ophthalmic Surg Lasers Imaging.* 2003;34(5):386–390. http://www.ncbi.nlm.nih.gov/pubmed/14509462.

66. Chen E, Lin MY, Cox J, Brown DM. Endophthalmitis after intravitreal injection: the importance of viridans streptococci. *Retina.* 2011;31(8):1525–1533. https://doi.org/10.1097/IAE.0b013e318221594a.

67. Diabetic Retinopathy Clinical Research Network (DRCR. net), Beck RW, Edwards AR, et al. Three-year follow-up of a randomized trial comparing focal/grid photocoagulation and intravitreal triamcinolone for diabetic macular edema. *Arch Ophthalmol.* 2009;127(3):245. https://doi.org/10.1001/archophthalmol.2008.610.

68. Nguyen QD, Brown DM, Marcus DM, et al. Ranibizumab for diabetic macular edema. *Ophthalmology.* 2012;119(4):789–801. https://doi.org/10.1016/j.ophtha.2011.12.039.

69. Diabetic Retinopathy Clinical Research Network, Wells JA, Glassman AR, et al. Aflibercept, bevacizumab, or ranibizumab for diabetic macular edema. *N Engl J Med.* 2015;372(13):1193–1203. https://doi.org/10.1056/NEJMoa1414264.

70. Gonzalez VH, Giuliari GP, Banda RM, Guel DA. Intravitreal injection of pegaptanib sodium for proliferative diabetic retinopathy. *Br J Ophthalmol.* 2009;93(11):1474–1478. https://doi.org/10.1136/bjo.2008.155663.

71. Gross JG, Glassman AR, Jampol LM, et al. Panretinal photocoagulation vs intravitreous ranibizumab for proliferative diabetic retinopathy. *JAMA.* 2015;314(20):2137. https://doi.org/10.1001/jama.2015.15217.

72. Mirshahi A, Roohipoor R, Lashay A, Mohammadi S-F, Abdoallahi A, Faghihi H. Bevacizumab-augmented retinal laser photocoagulation in proliferative diabetic retinopathy: a randomized double-masked clinical trial. *Eur J Ophthalmol.* 2018;18(2):263–269. http://www.ncbi.nlm.nih.gov/pubmed/18320520.

73. Zhang Z-H, Liu H-Y, Hernandez-Da Mota SE, et al. Vitrectomy with or without preoperative intravitreal bevacizumab for proliferative diabetic retinopathy: a meta-analysis of randomized controlled trials. *Am J Ophthalmol.* 2013;156(1):106–115.e2. https://doi.org/10.1016/j.ajo.2013.02.008.

74. Wu L, Martínez-Castellanos MA, Quiroz-Mercado H, et al. Twelve-month safety of intravitreal injections of bevacizumab (Avastin®): results of the Pan-American collaborative retina study group (PACORES). *Graefe's Arch Clin Exp Ophthalmol.* 2007;246(1):81–87. https://doi.org/10.1007/s00417-007-0660-z.

75. Day S, Acquah K, Mruthyunjaya P, Grossman DS, Lee PP, Sloan FA. Ocular complications after anti-vascular endothelial growth factor therapy in Medicare patients with age-related macular degeneration. *Am J Ophthalmol.* 2011;152(2):266–272. https://doi.org/10.1016/j.ajo.2011.01.053.

76. Mason JO, Frederick PA, Neimkin MG, et al. Incidence of hemorrhagic complications after intravitreal bevacizumab (avastin) or ranibizumab (lucentis) injections on systemically anticoagulated patients. *Retina.* 2010;30(9):1386–1389. https://doi.org/10.1097/IAE.0b013e3181e09739.

77. Baino F. Towards an ideal biomaterial for vitreous replacement: historical overview and future trends. *Acta Biomater.* 2011;7(3):921–935. https://doi.org/10.1016/j.actbio.2010.10.030.

78. Early vitrectomy for severe vitreous hemorrhage in diabetic retinopathy. Four-year results of a randomized trial: diabetic retinopathy vitrectomy study report 5. *Arch Ophthalmol (Chicago, Ill 1960).* 1990;108(7):958–964. http://www.ncbi.nlm.nih.gov/pubmed/2196036.

79. Early vitrectomy for severe proliferative diabetic retinopathy in eyes with useful vision. Results of a randomized trial–diabetic retinopathy vitrectomy study report 3. The diabetic retinopathy vitrectomy study research group. *Ophthalmology.* 1988;95(10):1307–1320. http://www.ncbi.nlm.nih.gov/pubmed/2465517.

80. Kralinger MT, Pedri M, Kralinger F, Troger J, Kieselbach GF. Long-term outcome after vitrectomy for diabetic macular edema. *Ophthalmologica.* 2006;220(3):147–152. https://doi.org/10.1159/000091756.

81. Stolba U, Binder S, Gruber D, Krebs I, Aggermann T, Neumaier B. Vitrectomy for persistent diffuse diabetic macular edema. *Am J Ophthalmol.* 2005;140(2):295–301. https://doi.org/10.1016/j.ajo.2005.03.045.

82. Boehm BO, Lang GK, Jehle PM, Feldman B, Lang GE. Octreotide reduces vitreous hemorrhage and loss of visual acuity risk in patients with high-risk proliferative diabetic retinopathy. *Horm Metab Res.* 2001;33(5):300–306. https://doi.org/10.1055/s-2001-15282.

83. Grant MB, Mames RN, Fitzgerald C, et al. The efficacy of octreotide in the therapy of severe nonproliferative and early proliferative diabetic retinopathy: a randomized controlled study. *Diabetes Care.* 2000;23(4):504–509. http://www.ncbi.nlm.nih.gov/pubmed/10857943.

84. Canonge RS, Bandello F, Ponsati B, et al. Topical administration of somatostatin and brimonidine in the early stages of diabetic retinopathy: results of the EUROCONDOR study. In: *EASD Virtual Meeting.* 2017:120.

85. Song JH, Chin HS, Kwon OW, Lim SJ, Kim HK. DRESS Research Group. Effect of sulodexide in patients with non-proliferative diabetic retinopathy: diabetic retinopathy sulodexide study (DRESS). *Graefes Arch Clin Exp Ophthalmol.* 2015;253(6):829–837. https://doi.org/10.1007/s00417-014-2746-8.

86. Campochiaro PA, Sophie R, Tolentino M, et al. Treatment of diabetic macular edema with an inhibitor of vascular endothelial-protein tyrosine phosphatase that activates Tie2. *Ophthalmology.* 2015;122(3):545–554. https://doi.org/10.1016/j.ophtha.2014.09.023.

87. Singerman L. Intravitreal bevasiranib in exudative age-related macular degeneration or diabetic macular edema. In: *Annual Meeting of the American Society of Retina Specialists.* 2007.

88. Boyer D, Quiroz-Mercado H, Kuppermann B, et al. Integrin peptide therapy: a new class of treatment for vascular eye diseases - the first human experience in DME. In: *ARVO.* 2012.

FURTHER READING

1. Early Treatment Diabetic Retinopathy Study Research Group. Grading diabetic retinopathy from stereoscopic color fundus photographs—an extension of the modified Airlie House classification: ETDRS report number 10. *Ophthalmology.* 1991;98:786–806.

2. Krein K, Skorin Jr L. Ocular manifestations of diabetes. *Consultant.* 2015;55(4):270–276.

CHAPTER 9

Depression and Type 2 DM in Adolescence

SHAKIRA F. SUGLIA, SCD, MS

INTRODUCTION

Depression (major *depressive* disorder or clinical *depression*) is a common but serious mood disorder that affects how people feel, think, and handle daily activities. Symptoms can include feelings of sadness, hopelessness, and loss of interest in daily activities that can affect daily functioning, such as sleeping, eating, attending school, and working. Severe symptoms can also include suicidal thoughts and attempted suicide. The prevalence of depression is highest among adults but also prevalent among children and adolescents. Rates of depression are higher among women compared to men in both childhood and adulthood. Depression is also associated with a number of chronic health conditions. Adults with depression are more likely to develop diabetes mellitus (DM) as well as insulin resistance.[1] Diagnosis of type 2 DM (T2DM) in adulthood has also been associated with depressive symptomatology and impaired quality of life,[1] suggesting a bidirectional association between T2DM and depression. Furthermore, among adults with T2DM, those with depression have a 1.5 times higher risk of morality, emphasizing the need to identify and treat depression among T2DM patients. Similar to findings among adults, recent evidence suggests the prevalence of depression among youth with T2DM to be higher compared to healthy youth, and some studies suggest among youth with both T2DM and depression the management of their illness to be more difficult.[2] Among youth, studies examining the comorbid prevalence of diabetes and depression, the consequences of this comorbid state or the examination into the mechanisms that may link diabetes and depression among youth are limited. The existing limited research in this area is summarized later as well as recommendations on future research endeavors and current clinical recommendations.

DEPRESSION AND T2DM AMONG YOUTH

The prevalence of depression among adolescents is high with some estimates suggesting 20% of adolescents experiencing at least one episode in their lifetime, with higher estimates among girls.[3] Adolescence is an important period of development because many health behaviors are established during these formative years.[4] Adolescent depression has been associated with overweight and obesity in adulthood,[5,6] and adolescent onset of depression is associated with both persistence of depression into adulthood and the development of other comorbid psychiatric disorders throughout the life course.[7] The prevalence of T2DM among youth has been on the rise partly attributed to the current obesity epidemic. Studies on the comorbidity of depression and diabetes largely come from studies examining youth with type 1 diabetes or obesity, noting a higher prevalence of depression and impaired quality of life among those with both chronic conditions.[8] These studies suggest youth onset of T2DM may be associated with emotional and behavioral complications resulting from the burden of managing a chronic condition.

Given that the occurrence of T2DM among children and adolescents has only been recently recognized there is a dearth of research examining its potential association with mental health outcomes, such as depression and T2DM in childhood and adolescence. The literature on the causes and consequences of childhood obesity that is more extensive has demonstrated that depression and depressive symptomatology are associated with childhood obesity suggesting that depression may also be associated with T2DM in childhood/adolescence. Only a handful of studies however have examined the association between depression or depression symptoms and T2DM among youth. In a study of primarily overweight/obese children within the Treatment Options for Type 2 Diabetes in Adolescents and Youth (TODAY) study, a

Pediatric Type II Diabetes. https://doi.org/10.1016/B978-0-323-55138-0.00009-7

cohort of youth with type 2 diabetes, rates of significant depressive symptoms were similar to those of healthy adolescents, however they were elevated among older girls in the cohort.[9] The prevalence of high depressive symptomatology among girls 16 years of age or older was 22% compared to 4% among boys of the same age. Other studies have examined these associations focusing on those at risk of developing T2DM, particularly youth who are obese. In a cross-sectional analysis of seventh graders at risk for developing T2DM who were participating in a school-based intervention to reduce obesity, depressive symptoms were associated with higher BMI and higher fasting insulin levels, consistent with the adult literature linking depression to clinical health markers.[10] In other work based on retrospective reports among youth attending an obesity clinic, Hannon and colleagues reported that those with higher scores on a depressive symptoms inventory had higher fasting insulin and Homeostatic model assessment for insulin resistance (HOMA-IR) values suggesting higher risk of T2DM among obese youth with high depressive symptomatology.[11] In a small study of children with familial history of early-onset type 2 diabetes, it was noted that depressive symptoms were common in children with a family history of early-onset type 2 diabetes and cooccurred with childhood diagnosis of type 2 diabetes. In fact, depressive symptoms score was predicted best by the number of generations of diabetes in the family.[12]

Only a few studies have examined the longitudinal relationship between adolescent mental health and the development of diabetes or the long-term impact of comorbid depression and diabetes on health and well-being. Among children at risk for developing obesity and diabetes in adulthood, Shomaker and colleagues examined the relation between childhood depressive symptomatology and insulin resistance 6 years after the childhood depressive symptoms assessment.[13] Children's depressive symptoms were associated with follow-up HOMA-IR, fasting insulin, and fasting glucose in models accounting for baseline HOMA-IR, insulin or glucose value, baseline BMI and changes in BMI as well as demographic factors and family history of T2DM, suggesting that depressive symptoms can alter insulin resistance independent of changes in BMI during child and adolescent development. Although mechanism for this association was not explored the authors suggest decreases in energy expenditure as well as emotional eating patterns that may cause weight gain., However, the authors did adjust for changes in BMI suggesting that other mechanisms may be responsible for the noted associations. It is also hypothesized that depressive symptoms promote insulin resistance by upregulating cortisol however this association has not been examined among children or adolescents. A handful of studies has furthermore examined the longitudinal association between depressive symptoms in adolescence and development of T2DM in adulthood. For example, in a large study based on the 1946 British Cohort Study, adolescent affective disorder was associated with DM at age 53.[14] Using data from the National Longitudinal Study of Adolescent to Adult Health (Add Health) a nationally representative cohort of US adolescents, the relationship of depression symptoms during adolescence and young adulthood with the development of T2DM in adulthood was examined. The incidence of T2DM varied by the presence of depression symptoms (Table 9.1). Among women who did not experience high levels of depressive symptoms in either adolescence or adulthood, the incidence of T2DM was 3.0%; among women who experienced high levels of depressive symptoms in adolescence, adulthood, or both, it ranged from 4.1% to 7.5%. Among men who did not experience high levels of depressive symptoms, the incidence of T2DM was 3.3%. The incidence of T2DM among men who experienced high levels of depressive symptoms varied: Men with high levels of depressive symptoms in adolescence only had the highest incidence of T2DM, at 4.3%, and those who experienced high levels of depressive symptoms in both adolescence and adulthood had the lowest incidence of T2DM, at 2.0%. In adjusted analyses, women were at a higher risk of developing T2DM if they experienced high levels of depressive symptoms during both adolescence and adulthood (odds ratio = 1.96, 95% confidence interval: 1.23, 3.11) than were those who did not experience a high level of symptoms at either time point. No statistically significant associations were noted among men (odds ratio = 0.46, 95% confidence interval: 0.20, 1.05). These findings suggest that the onset of depression early in life may set up a trajectory of risk for development of DM among women. Factors that influence adult DM, such as depression, may originate in childhood and adolescence and influence the trajectory of DM development.

Other studies have focused on youth with T2DM and depressive symptoms. Lawrence and colleagues noted higher levels of depressed mood to be associated with poor glycemic control and number of emergency department visits among participants with both T1DM and T2DM, compared with youth with T1DM and T2DM who had low levels of depressed mood.[15] Among children enrolled in the Pediatric Diabetes Consortium T1D and T2D registries, depressive symptomatology was common in T1D participants, but the prevalence of

TABLE 9.1
Incidence of T2DM in Adulthood by Depressive Symptomatology in Adolescence and Adulthood, Add Health Study

| Depression Category and Timing[a] | INCIDENCE OF TYPE 2 DIABETES MELLITUS | | | | | |
| | MEN (n = 6032) | | | WOMEN (n = 6625) | | |
	No.[b]	%	SE	No.[b]	%	SE
Low	172	3.31	0.4	171	3.04	0.3
High in adolescence only	31	4.34	1.1	60	4.51	0.8
High in adulthood only	22	3.89	1.3	33	4.09	1.1
High in adolescence and adulthood	10	2.03	0.9	53	7.51	1.4

SE, standard error.
[a]High levels of depressive symptoms were defined as a score on the Center for Epidemiologic Studies Depression Scale of 16 or higher on the 20-item version (administered to the sample during adolescence) or 11 or higher on the 10-item version (used in the wave 4 follow-up interview in adulthood).
[b]Sample size of study participants with type 2 diabetes mellitus, unweighted.
Taken with permission from Suglia SF, Demmer RT, Wahi R, Keyes KM, Koenen KC. Depressive symptoms during adolescence and young adulthood and the development of type 2 diabetes mellitus. *Am J Epidemiol.* 2016; 183:269–276.

depressive symptoms was nearly twofold higher in youth with T2D.[16] These findings are consistent with those of the SEARCH study where a higher prevalence of depressive symptoms in adolescents with type 1 diabetes vs youth in the general population was also reported.[17]

CLINICAL IMPLICATIONS

The American Academy of Pediatrics recommends the screening and management of depression in its report "Management of Type 2 Diabetes Mellitus in Children and Adolescents".[18] The report acknowledges the lack of longitudinal studies of the association between T2DM and depression among youth. However, given existing evidence from cross-sectional studies on the prevalence of depressive symptomatology among youth with T2DM and its association with poor glycemic control, number of Emergency Departments (ED) visits, and overall poor adherence to therapeutic treatment it is recommended that clinicians screen youth with T2DM for depression at diagnosis and that periodic routine screening is performed particularly among those with frequent ED visits and/or poor glycemic control.[18] Positive screening for depression should be followed with referral to a mental health provider. Furthermore, the American Academy of Pediatrics has recently updated their recommendations regarding the screening, diagnosis, and initial management of depression among youth ages 10–21 and recommends annual screening for depression for all youth 12 years of age or older.[3] This recommendation is in accordance with the United

States Preventive Services Task Force guidelines, which also recommends screening for depression among adolescents 12–18 years of age.[19] There is no single intervention that will treat depression in adolescents with T2D. However, family, peer support, and an organized and simplified care plan are key to positive diabetes self-management and adherence.

Research Recommendations

As noted, cross-sectional studies note a higher prevalence of depression among youth at risk for T2DM or with diagnosed T1DM or T2DM. There is however a dearth of research that examines the relation between depression and T2DM across the life course or that focuses on potential modifiers, including those that may increase vulnerability or have a salutary effect.

Need for longitudinal studies. Because risk factors and health behaviors known to affect obesity and diabetes can persist from childhood to adolescence and into adulthood, a life-course framework for studying the relation between depression and T2DM is crucial. Reliance on assessments in adulthood of both depression and T2DM has limited the ability of investigators in most studies to address temporality, which raises the possibility of reverse causation, in which subclinical T2DM risk factors contribute to both depression and clinical T2DM development later in life.

Gender as a modifier of vulnerability. Although gender-specific risks among adults have been suggested in other studies, there are a limited number of studies in which gender differences in depression and diabetes among younger populations have been examined.[20] Among adolescents, there is evidence of a gender-differentiated association between depression and obesity. For example, in a study conducted among adolescents in New Zealand, Richardson et al.[6] noted that depression in adolescence was associated with obesity in adulthood among girls only. Different coping mechanisms among men and women have been proposed as explanations for gender differences in the development of metabolic disorders. However, previous analyses in which behavioral factors in adolescence and adulthood have been examined suggest a relationship between weight status, health behaviors (sleep duration, physical activity level, smoking status, and alcohol consumption), and depression that is similar across genders and therefore not likely to account for previously observed differences. Physiological mechanisms (e.g., hypothalamic-pituitary-adrenal axis dysregulation, inflammatory processes) that may account for noted gender differences in the relation between depression and DM are plausible and should be investigated in future studies.

Protective factors/Interventions. Currently, it is unknown what factors may mitigate the impact of depression on insulin resistance and risk of T2DM. It is also unknown whether pharmacologic or psychotherapeutic interventions that alleviate depression symptoms have a salutatory effect on insulin resistance, risk of T2DM or management of T2DM. Among adults with T2DM, positive psychological characteristics such as optimism, resilience, and self-esteem have been associated with lower mortality rates, improved glycemic controls and fewer complications.[21] Whether these factors could have an impact on at-risk youth or youth with T2DM is unknown but presents a future area of research that may inform intervention efforts.

CONCLUSIONS

Given the high prevalence of depression among adolescents and the increased prevalence of T2DM among youth in the past recent years, a continued focus on depression and its association with T2DM is warranted. Future works should focus on how depression may affect the development of T2DM and management of T2DM. More investigation is essential to explore how youth with T2DM may be at greater risk for developing depression and what interventions (i.e., medications, nutrition, exercise, or resiliency) may ameliorate the consequences of experiencing these comorbid conditions.

REFERENCES

1. Kan C, Silva N, Golden SH, et al. A systematic review and meta-analysis of the association between depression and insulin resistance. *Diabetes Care*. 2013;36(2):480–489.
2. Stewart SM, Rao U, White P. Depression and diabetes in children and adolescents. *Curr Opin Pediatr*. 2005;17(5):626–631.
3. Zuckerbrot RA, Cheung A, Jensen PS, Stein REK, Laraque D, Glad PC, Steering G. Guidelines for adolescent depression in primary care (GLAD-PC): part I. Practice preparation, identification, assessment, and initial management. *Pediatrics*. 2018.
4. Nolen-Hoeksema S. *Sex Differences in Depression*. Stanford, CA: Stanford University Press; 1990.
5. Frisco ML, Houle JN, Lippert AM. Weight change and depression among US young women during the transition to adulthood. *Am J Epidemiol*. 2013;178(1):22–30.
6. Richardson LP, Davis R, Poulton R, et al. A longitudinal evaluation of adolescent depression and adult obesity. *Archiv Pediatr Adolesc Med*. 2003;157(8):739–745.
7. Pine DS, Cohen E, Cohen P, Brook J. Adolescent depressive symptoms as predictors of adult depression: moodiness or mood disorder? *Am J Psychiat*. 1999;156(1):133–135.
8. Buchberger B, Huppertz H, Krabbe L, Lux B, Mattivi JT, Siafarikas A. Symptoms of depression and anxiety in youth with type 1 diabetes: a systematic review and meta-analysis. *Psychoneuroendocrinology*. 2016;70:70–84.
9. Anderson BJ, Edelstein S, Abramson NW, et al. Depressive symptoms and quality of life in adolescents with type 2 diabetes: baseline data from the TODAY study. *Diabetes Care*. 2011;34(10):2205–2207.
10. Jaser SS, Holl MG, Jefferson V, Grey M. Correlates of depressive symptoms in urban youth at risk for type 2 diabetes mellitus. *J Sch Health*. 2009;79(6):286–292.
11. Hannon TS, Li Z, Tu W, et al. Depressive symptoms are associated with fasting insulin resistance in obese youth. *Pediatr Obes*. 2014;9(5):e103–e107.
12. Irving RR, Mills JL, Choo-Kang EG, et al. Diabetes and psychological co-morbidity in children with a family history of early-onset type 2 diabetes. *Int J Psychol*. 2008;43(6):937–942.
13. Shomaker LB, Tanofsky-Kraff M, Stern EA, et al. Longitudinal study of depressive symptoms and progression of insulin resistance in youth at risk for adult obesity. *Diabetes Care*. 2011;34(11):2458–2463.
14. Gaysina D, Pierce M, Richards M, Hotopf M, Kuh D, Hardy R. Association between adolescent emotional problems and metabolic syndrome: the modifying effect of C-reactive protein gene (CRP) polymorphisms. *Brain Behav Immun*. 2011;25(4):750–758.
15. Lawrence JM, Standiford DA, Loots B, et al. Prevalence and correlates of depressed mood among youth with diabetes: the SEARCH for Diabetes in Youth study. *Pediatrics*. 2006;117(4):1348–1358.

16. Silverstein J, Cheng P, Ruedy KJ, et al. Depressive symptoms in youth with type 1 or type 2 diabetes: results of the pediatric diabetes consortium screening assessment of depression in diabetes study. *Diabetes Care.* 2015;38(12):2341–2343.
17. Hood KK, Beavers DP, Yi-Frazier J, et al. Psychosocial burden and glycemic control during the first 6 years of diabetes: results from the SEARCH for Diabetes in Youth study. *J Adolesc Health.* 2014;55(4):498–504.
18. Springer SC, Silverstein J, Copeland K, et al. Management of type 2 diabetes mellitus in children and adolescents. *Pediatrics.* 2013;131(2):e648–e664.
19. Forman-Hoffman V, McClure E, McKeeman J, et al. Screening for major depressive disorder in children and adolescents: a systematic review for the U.S. Preventive Services Task Force. *Ann Intern Med.* 2016;164(5):342–349.
20. Kumari M, Head J, Marmot M. Prospective study of social and other risk factors for incidence of type 2 diabetes in the Whitehall II study. *Archiv Intern Med.* 2004;164(17):1873–1880.
21. Celano CM, Beale EE, Moore SV, Wexler DJ, Huffman JC. Positive psychological characteristics in diabetes: a review. *Curr Diab Rep.* 2013;13(6):917–929.

CHAPTER 10

PCOS and Type II Diabetes

MARISSA AVOLIO, MD • HEBA M. ISMAIL, MBBCH, MSC, PHD

INTRODUCTION

Polycystic ovary syndrome (PCOS) is a common, multifactorial endocrinopathy. An estimated 5%–20% of young women are afflicted with the syndrome, depending upon the diagnostic criteria used and the ethnic population being studied, although general prevalence in the adult population is quoted to be 4%–6%.[1,2] In the 1980s, insulin resistance (IR) and a resulting increased risk for type 2 diabetes (T2D) were recognized as important complications of the disease.[3] Three studies published in the late 1990s and early 2000s looking at large cross-sectional cohorts of lean and obese women with PCOS in the United States (US) estimated the prevalence of impaired glucose tolerance (IGT) to be 23%–35%, with an additional 4%–10% of the women having T2D; a much higher incidence of IGT and T2D than was found in controls. In adolescents, Palmert et al. looked at IR and dysglycemia among girls with PCOS.[4] They showed that these disorders were also common in this younger population, with one third of the 27 girls studied showing evidence of abnormal glucose tolerance by oral glucose tolerance test (OGTT), eight having IGT, and one fulfilling criteria for diagnosis of diabetes.

PATHOPHYSIOLOGY

PCOS arises from a combination of genetic and environmental factors. Although no single gene has been identified as causative, genome-wide association studies (GWAS) have discovered multiple susceptibility loci.[1,5] Additionally, the disease tends to run in families, with women whose mothers or sisters have been diagnosed with PCOS having up to a 50% risk of being diagnosed with the disorder themselves.[1]

Although not all of the pathogenesis details have been worked out, it is believed that dysregulated gonadotropin secretion and ovarian androgen overproduction are major contributors to the PCOS phenotype (Fig. 10.1). Females with this disease have higher luteinizing hormone (LH) secretion, which stimulates theca cells to produce larger quantities of androstenedione. Androstenedione, in turn, serves as a substrate for 17β hydroxysteroid dehydrogenase, and is converted to testosterone. Elevated androgens then create many of the symptoms young women find most distressing, including hirsutism, acne, and alopecia. Meanwhile, high circulating insulin levels from inherent insulin resistance, which is only worsened by obesity and puberty, stimulate LH production, pushing the ovaries to produce more androgens. The elevated LH and insulin levels work in conjunction with one another to cause polycystic ovaries, and without follicular maturation, affected adolescents and women become anovulatory.[6] Although the vast majority of hyperandrogenism arises from the ovaries, up to one third of patients may also exhibit elevations in adrenal androgens, especially dehydroepiandrosterone-sulfate (DHEA-S).[2]

ROLE OF INSULIN IN ANDROGEN EXCESS

As mentioned earlier, PCOS is associated with ovarian hyperandrogenism. In addition to LH, it has been suggested that insulin and insulin-like growth factor-1 (IGF-1) also stimulate the theca cells to produce androgens.[3,7,8] As a result of the patients' insulin resistance, hyperinsulinemia is observed, which in turn stimulates LH and ovarian androgen production, thus worsening hyperandrogenemia.[9] Interestingly, LH-producing cells in the pituitary and ovarian theca cells seem to preserve their sensitivity to insulin in PCOS, despite most tissues in the body becoming insulin resistant.[7] Higher insulin levels also lower sex hormone binding globulin (SHBG) by halting its production in the liver, allowing for the circulation of greater quantities of unbound androgens, enhancing granulosa and theca cell sensitivity to LH, and further promoting ovarian steroid production.[1,10] It has been postulated that there is also an intrinsic ovarian defect that contributes to hyperandrogenism, as theca cells from PCOS patients grown in

Pediatric Type II Diabetes. https://doi.org/10.1016/B978-0-323-55138-0.00010-3
Copyright © 2019 Elsevier Inc. All rights reserved.

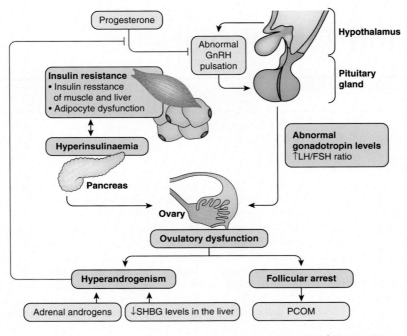

Nature Reviews | Disease Primers

FIG. 10.1 The pathophysiology of PCOS. *FSH*, follicle stimulating hormone; *GnRH*, gonadotropin releasing hormone; *LH*, luteinizing hormone; *SHBG*, sex hormone binding globulin. (From Azziz R, Carmina E, Chen Z, et al. Polycystic ovary syndrome. Nature reviews. *Disease Primers*. 2016;2:16057. https://doi.org/10.1038/nrdp.2016.57. [published Online First: Epub Date], with permission.)

media lacking LH continue to hypersecrete androgens when stimulated with either LH or insulin.[11]

DIAGNOSIS/CLASSIFICATION OF PCOS

The diagnosis of PCOS is not standardized, although hyperandrogenism and ovulatory dysfunction have been agreed upon as central to the disease. In 1990, the National Institute of Child Health and Human Development (NICHD) branch of the National Institutes of Health (NIH) sponsored a conference where experts met and voted to determine a formal definition for the diagnosis of PCOS. They settled upon chronic anovulation with evidence of hyperandrogenism on examination or laboratory evaluation that cannot be attributed to another source.[3] In 2003, experts from the European Society for Human Reproduction and the American Society for Reproductive Medicine met in Rotterdam, and devised guidelines that accounted for the wider spectrum of phenotypes observed in clinical practice. Having ruled out other etiologies, two of three criteria, oligo- and/or anovulation, clinical and/or biochemical

hyperandrogenism, and polycystic ovaries, were determined to be diagnostic of PCOS.[3,12] Then, in 2006, the Androgen Excess and PCOS Society task force published their recommendations on diagnosing PCOS, based on the available literature. Their guidelines focused on the diagnosis being rooted in hyperandrogenism with accompanying ovarian dysfunction. They described nine phenotypes characteristic of PCOS, and incorporated the recognition of associated comorbidities, including obesity, insulin resistance, and hyperinsulinism into their discussion of the disease.[13]

Six years later, in 2012, the NIH convened for an evidence based methodology workshop on PCOS, where they evaluated the criteria that had been put forth thus far.[14] They recommended utilizing the Rotterdam criteria, with emphasis on classification into four phenotypes (androgen excess + ovulatory dysfunction, androgen excess + polycystic ovarian morphology, ovulatory dysfunction + polycystic ovarian morphology, and androgen excess + ovulatory dysfunction + polycystic ovarian morphology). The Endocrine Society followed with their PCOS Clinical Practice Guidelines the following year.[15] They utilized the Rotterdam criteria for diagnosing PCOS, but did qualify that certain abnormalities seen in adult women are part of normal pubertal progression, thereby acknowledging that diagnosing adolescents with PCOS is different.

Diagnosis of PCOS in adolescence presents particular challenges. It is common for teenagers to experience irregular menses and anovulatory cycles for at least 2 years, and, less commonly, up to 6 years after menarche.[15] Furthermore, polycystic ovaries can be a normal finding in youths, and it is rare to progress through puberty without acne, a clinical sign of hyperandrogenism in adults.[15] Therefore, members from the Androgen Excess-PCOS society in conjunction with some of their international colleagues published a paper clarifying the criteria for PCOS diagnosis in the teenage years.[16] In it, they recommended that significant hirsutism be regarded as a sign of hyperandrogenism, and that patients with difficult to treat acne have androgen levels drawn. Elevations in total or free testosterone are to be present on more than one lab draw. Absence of menstrual cycles for greater than 90 days at any time after menarche, as well as failure to achieve menarche by age 15 years or beyond 2–3 years from breast development, were all felt to warrant workup for oligomenorrhea. Ovarian imaging was considered unnecessary in adolescents, and caution was recommended against making a diagnosis of PCOS without at least 2 years of oligomenorrhea.[16] Finally, it should be emphasized that IR and T2D do not play a role in diagnosing PCOS, as evidenced by their omission from all of the diagnostic criteria and classifications referenced earlier.

It is important to remember that PCOS is a diagnosis of exclusion. Although more common than most of these, other causes of menstrual irregularities, obesity, and/or hyperandrogenism including nonclassical congenital adrenal hyperplasia (CAH), androgen secreting adrenal or ovarian tumors, primary pigmented nodular adrenocortical disease, McCune Albright syndrome, Cushing's syndrome, thyroid dysfunction, hyperprolactinemia, acromegaly, glucocorticoid resistance secondary to glucocorticoid receptor gene mutations, hypogonadism, and idiopathic hirsutism should all be considered prior to diagnosing PCOS.[12,13,16,17]

INSULIN RESISTANCE

In 1997, the American Diabetes Association (ADA) defined insulin resistance as "an impaired biological response to either exogenous or endogenous insulin."[18] Insulin resistance is measured using hyperinsulinemic-euglycemic clamp studies, which are capable of

identifying "impaired insulin stimulated glucose disposal," and may also be defined as the "lowest quartile of measures of insulin sensitivity (i.e., insulin stimulated glucose uptake during hyperinsulinemic-euglycemic clamp) for the background population under investigation."[2] Given the time, expense, and invasive nature of clamp studies, estimations of insulin resistance using labs from a single blood draw such as the homeostatic model assessment of β-cell function and insulin resistance (HOMA-IR) have also been devised.[19]

Although IR is not part of the clinical criteria for diagnosing PCOS, studies suggest that over 80% of patients may develop it.[9] Adult PCOS patients have a relative risk of 1.95 of being overweight and 2.77 of being obese compared to women without the disease.[20] Similarly, adolescent girls who are overweight to very obese have been found to have odds ratios of 2.95–14.65 of carrying a diagnosis of PCOS when compared to girls who are underweight or of a normal weight.[21] Nonetheless, PCOS patients tend to be insulin resistant independent of their weight, and despite weight loss or antiandrogenic therapy.[1–3,7,9,22] A meta-analysis of 28 hyperinsulinemic-euglycemic clamp studies conducted in women with PCOS (diagnosed by either NIH or Rotterdam criteria) between 18 and 40 years of age showed that PCOS is associated with a 27% lower insulin sensitivity, independent of BMI. When BMI was factored in, it was estimated to lower insulin sensitivity by an additional 15%. The effect of obesity on insulin resistance was greater in PCOS patients than in controls.[23]

Studies using IV glucose tolerance testing (IVGTT) have found that 53%–76% of Hispanic and non-Hispanic American, southern Italian, and Japanese women with PCOS meet criteria for insulin resistance.[24,25] A euglycemic clamp study demonstrated that 26% of obese patients with PCOS, and 60% of non-obese patients with PCOS exhibited insulin stimulated glucose usage that was less than that of weight matched subjects without PCOS.[22] Hepatic glucose production could not be suppressed in 26.7% of the obese patients with PCOS, and in 20% of the nonobese PCOS patients, with complete suppression in all of the patients without PCOS.[22]

The trend of insulin resistance is seen in adolescents as well, and is amplified by the physiologic increase in growth hormone that occurs during this period of rapid growth and development.[26] When 12 young girls with PCOS and 10 age-matched obese controls underwent hyperinsulinemic-euglycemic and hyperglycemic clamps to assess insulin sensitivity and insulin secretion, the girls with PCOS were found to have significantly higher insulin levels, 50% lower peripheral insulin sensitivity, as well as evidence of hepatic insulin resistance.[27] Another study performed IVGTTs on 13 girls (ages 11–18 years) with hyperandrogenism in the form of hirsutism with or without acne and acanthosis, and most with menstrual irregularity, as well as 28 girls without these symptoms. Only two of the controls were obese, compared to six of the girls with hyperandrogenism. Fasting insulin levels were significantly higher in the girls with hyperandrogenism versus controls (256 ± 35 vs. 103 ± 24 pmol/L, P = .0008). Additionally, it took longer for glucose levels to fall from their peak in the girls with hyperandrogenism than it did in the controls (40.8 ± 2.7 min compared to 33.1 ± 2.2 min, P = .03).[28]

Being born small for gestational age (SGA), particularly when followed by rapid catch up growth, is a risk factor for PCOS, insulin resistance, development of central obesity, and even early puberty.[7] Studies have identified greater insulin resistance in both 1 year old and 9 year old children who were born SGA when compared to their peers born at appropriate birth weights.[29,30] Excess weight also confers risk, as females who are large for gestational age (LGA) carry a higher risk of hyperandrogenemia and PCOS than their normal weight counterparts, and girls who are obese during late childhood have elevated testosterone and insulin levels as they progress through puberty.[31–33]

Premature adrenarche in girls is also a known marker for increased likelihood of IR and of developing PCOS.[8] As part of a study by Ibáñez et al.,[8] 10 girls with PCOS and a history of premature pubarche underwent OGTTs. None of the subjects were obese, and all had evidence of hyperinsulinemia, with eight showing higher insulin levels as far back as their premature pubarche diagnosis.

In addition to being insulin resistant, women with PCOS of any weight have been found to secrete less insulin than necessary for their degree of insulin resistance, suggestive of intrinsic β-cell dysfunction.[2,34] Insulin measurements following frequently sampled IVGTTs, graded increases in IV glucose infusions, and oscillatory glucose boluses over a 16-h period in 24 obese women with PCOS were compared to those of eight women without the diagnosis.[35] Although those with PCOS had normal first phase insulin responses to the IVGTT and graded glucose infusions, the women with a family history of T2D were noted to have decreased insulin secretion when their degree of insulin resistance was accounted for. Furthermore, these women's pancreases were unable to appropriately adapt to the oscillatory glucose boluses, concerning for β-cell impairment.[35]

The insulin receptor is a tyrosine kinase receptor comprised of two αβ heterodimers. Insulin binding to the extracellular α subunit promotes autophosphorylation. This then activates the β-subunit's tyrosine kinase,

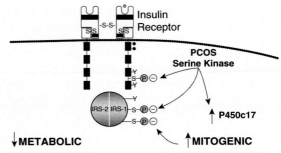

FIG. 10.2 Proposed insulin-signaling defects in PCOS. (From Diamanti-Kandarakis E, Dunaif A. Insulin resistance and the polycystic ovary syndrome revisited: an update on mechanisms and implications. *Endocr Rev*. 2012;33(6):981–1030. https://doi.org/10.1210/er.2011-1034. [published Online First: Epub Date], with permission.)

causing phosphorylation of tyrosine residues on insulin receptor substrates (IRS), which in turn bind targets including phosphatidylinositol 3-kinase (PI3-K), causing downstream signal transduction that leads to movement of the GLUT4 glucose transporter to the cell surface, promotion of glycogen and protein synthesis, and inhibition of lipolysis.[34] Studies conducted in the fibroblasts and adipocytes of women with PCOS have not found a deficiency in insulin receptors or differences in the receptor's binding.[36–39] However, adipocytes have been shown to be insulin resistant, take up significantly less glucose (perhaps the result of fewer GLUT4 transporters), and have less lipoprotein lipase activity.[3,34]

Several mechanisms have been proposed to explain the insulin resistance seen at the molecular level. Fibroblasts and skeletal muscle cells have demonstrated higher serine phosphorylation, yielding lower tyrosine kinase activity, which in turn decreases PI3-K activation, thus preventing the downstream cascade and possibly explaining the PCOS-induced insulin resistance.[3,34] The MAPK-ERK 1/2 mitogenic pathway has kinases which serine phosphorylate IRS-1. Studies using skeletal muscle of PCOS patients provide evidence of constitutive activation of this pathway, suggesting a contributing mechanism for insulin resistance in these women.[3] Cytochrome P450c17 is believed to be an important enzyme in androgen production that is activated by serine phosphorylation (Fig. 10.2). It has been proposed that a protein kinase that acts on both cytochrome P450c17 and IRS-1 would increase androgen production, while at the same time worsening insulin resistance, although one that fits this description has not yet been identified.[3]

Insulin resistance has also been attributed to high levels of free fatty acids (FFA), which have been demonstrated in women with PCOS.[3,34] Free fatty acids inhibit PI3-K activity by affecting IRS-1 phosphorylation, and inducing insulin resistance.[40] These defects and resulting insulin resistance occur when FFAs are infused into subjects, even without glucose tolerance concerns.[41] FFAs are also known to promote hepatic gluconeogenesis.[42]

An association between decreased adiponectin and increased plasminogen activator inhibitor-1 has also been made with insulin resistance.[5] Low adiponectin levels in obese women with PCOS were inversely correlated with BMI, testosterone, and insulin resistance.[5] GWAS and linkage studies looking at the adiponectin gene found single nucleotide polymorphisms that increase obesity, T2D, IR, and cardiovascular disease. These seem to occur more frequently in women diagnosed with PCOS, further supporting this connection.[9]

In conclusion, IR plays an important role in PCOS, affecting both adults and adolescents with the disease, independent of obesity. Females born SGA, LGA, or who experience premature adrenarche seem to be at greater risk for developing IR, and there are studies to suggest that despite their high insulin production, women with PCOS produce inadequate amounts of insulin for their degree of IR. At the molecular level, phosphorylation patterns of the insulin receptor and its targets appear to affect cell signaling in PCOS.

TYPE 2 DIABETES

It has been estimated that women with PCOS are 5–10 times more likely to develop T2D than the general population, with IR being an intrinsic part of the disease process.[2,3] Impaired glucose tolerance has been found to affect 30%–45% of obese PCOS patients, and 5%–15% carry a diagnosis of T2D.[9,10] About 2% of patients with PCOS without glucose abnormalities are estimated to develop T2D each year, while that number increases substantially to 16% in PCOS patients with IGT.[1]

One study evaluated 254 Caucasian women with PCOS (ages 14–44 years) with 2-h OGTTs, and showed that 31.1% had IGT. Although only 3.2% would have been diagnosed with T2D using ADA criteria, 7.5% fulfilled the World Health Organization (WHO) criteria (Fig. 10.3). It is of note that 73% of the subjects were obese, and 10% of the women between 25 and 35 years of age were afflicted with T2D, but this increased to 21% in those between 35 and 40 years of age.[2,43]

A second more diverse study looked at OGTTs from 122 Caucasian, non-Hispanic Black, Asian, and Hispanic PCOS patients. Thirty-five percent of subjects had IGT, and 10% met WHO criteria for T2D. Twenty-five

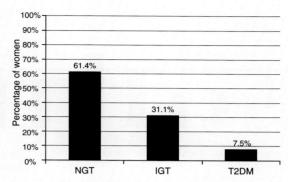

FIG. 10.3 Prevalence of normal glucose tolerance, impaired glucose tolerance, and type 2 diabetes by 1985 WHO criteria. *IGT*, impaired glucose tolerance; *NGT*, normal glucose tolerance; *T2DM*, type 2 diabetes mellitus. (From Ovalle F, Azziz R. Insulin resistance, polycystic ovary syndrome, and type 2 diabetes mellitus. *Fertil Steril*. 2002;77(6):1095–1105, with permission.)

of the patients who had normal baseline glucose tolerance were followed for up to 75 months, five of whom (20%) developed IGT, while one (4%) progressed to diabetes. Repeat OGTTs in 14 women who initially had IGT showed continued impairment in seven, normal glucose tolerance (NGT) in three, and diabetes in the remaining four. Family history of T2D was present in 83% of the patients who themselves were diagnosed with diabetes, 56% who had IGT, and 31% with NGT.[44]

A study of 239 women with PCOS between the ages of 20 and 40 years in Sarajevo[45] also examined OGTT changes over time. Ninety-one women (38%) had previously diagnosed T2D. Eighteen were diagnosed with prediabetes via initial OGTT, and five went on to develop T2D within 3 years' time. Forty-seven (36%) of the remaining 130 patients who did not have prediabetes during that first OGTT developed impaired fasting glucose (IFG) or IGT in 3 years. The women with the highest CRP, HOMA-IR, BMI, DHEA-S, and lipid accumulation product (a marker of insulin resistance that takes into account triglyceride levels and waist circumference), as well as the lowest 25-OH vitamin D levels were the most likely to become prediabetic. Women with elevated BMIs (18%) were more likely to be diagnosed with prediabetes than normal weight women (4%).[45]

A study in Finland[46] followed 5899 women born in 1966 through 46 years of age, with information available on glucose tolerance in 2841 of them. The 279 with PCOS (oligoamenorrhea and hirsutism by questionnaire at 31 years of age or having received an official diagnosis by 46 years old) were much more likely

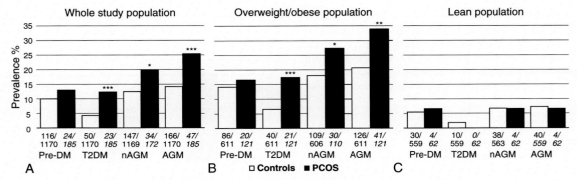

FIG. 10.4 Prevalence of prediabetes, type 2 diabetes, and abnormal glucose metabolism in women with PCOS compared to controls. **(A):** All patients in the study, **(B):** Patients with BMI>25 kg/m², **(C):** Patients with BMI<25 kg/m². *AGM,* abnormal glucose metabolism (prediabetes or type 2 diabetes); *nAGM,* new abnormal glucose metabolism (impaired fasting glucose, impaired glucose tolerance, or type 2 diabetes) picked up on OGTT at 46 years of age; *Pre-DM,* prediabetes; *T2DM,* type 2 diabetes. (From Ollila ME, West S, Keinanen-Kiukaanniemi S, et al. Overweight and obese but not normal weight women with PCOS are at increased risk of Type 2 diabetes mellitus-a prospective, population-based cohort study. *Hum Reprod (Oxf Engl).* 2017;32(2):423–431. https://doi.org/10.1093/humrep/dew329. [published Online First: Epub Date], with permission.)

to have abnormal glucose tolerance and T2D by WHO criteria than those without PCOS. Normal weight women (BMI≤25 kg/m²) with PCOS, however, were more likely to have normal glucose tolerance (only 6.5% of them had abnormal glucose tolerance, none of whom were diagnosed with T2D) than the heavier women with PCOS, and did not show a higher risk of glucose abnormalities compared to women without PCOS. Of the women with PCOS and a BMI greater than 25 kg/m² who developed T2D, 82.6% of them were diagnosed with T2D prior to age 46. Those who had PCOS and ultimately developed abnormal glucose tolerance were already heavier than their peers by age 14 years, and gained an average of 27.25 kg between 14 and 31 years of age compared to a weight gain of about 13.8 kg during the same time period in the women with normal glucose tolerance (Figs. 10.4 and 10.5).

Finally, a study of postmenopausal women found that 15% of those who carried a diagnosis of PCOS had T2D as opposed to only 2.3% of women of the same age without PCOS, signifying that glucose abnormalities may be maintained through much of the PCOS patients' lives.[47]

Researchers have also attempted to estimate the prevalence of abnormal glucose tolerance in adolescents with PCOS. In 2016, Coles et al. [48] published a retrospective chart review of Canadian teenagers with PCOS (with clinical or biochemical hyperandrogenism plus oligomenorrhea) who had had OGTTs to determine the prevalence of, and risk factors for, dysglycemia.

Glucose abnormalities were diagnosed based on the Canadian Diabetes Association 2013 Clinical Practice Guidelines, which are similar to the WHO cutoffs used for dysglycemia and T2D. The girls had a mean age of 15.4 years, and were over 3 years post-menarche. One hundred sixty-three of the patients had OGTT data, which revealed IGT in 26 (16%) and provisional T2D in 2 (1.2%), giving an overall prevalence of 17.2% of PCOS patients with dysglycemia. They also noted that the fasting glucose level was only abnormal in 2 of the 28 patients. The adolescents with glucose abnormalities had significantly higher BMI z-score and triglyceride levels. All of the patients with dysglycemia fell into the overweight or obese categories, and the obese girls were also more likely to report a family history of components of the metabolic syndrome, T2D, PCOS, or heart disease (P=.008).[48]

The use of HbA1c to aid in the diagnosis of glucose abnormalities in this population has also been explored. A study of 68 adolescents with PCOS by NIH criteria followed at Boston Children's Hospital (without previously diagnosed dysglycemia) looked retrospectively at OGTT and HbA1c data closest to the patients' PCOS diagnosis. OGTTs and HbA1c measurements had been done within 3 months of one another, although occurred on the same day in 66% of patients. Twenty-four patients had HbA1c levels greater than 5.6%. Three patients had IFG, and nine had IGT, while only one was diagnosed with diabetes using ADA criteria (this patient also had a diabetic range HbA1c).

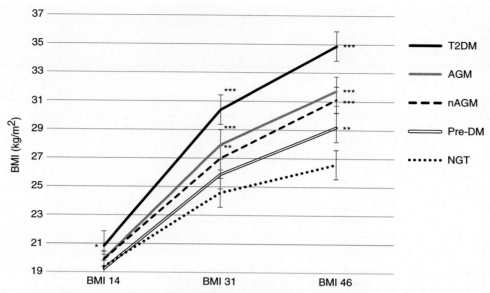

FIG. 10.5 Progression of BMI throughout life based on glucose metabolism status at 46 years of age. *AGM*, abnormal glucose metabolism (prediabetes or type 2 diabetes); *nAGM*, new abnormal glucose metabolism (impaired fasting glucose, impaired glucose tolerance, or type 2 diabetes) picked up on OGTT at 46 years of age; *NGT*, normal glucose tolerance; *Pre-DM*, prediabetes; *T2DM*, type 2 diabetes. (From Ollila ME, West S, Keinanen-Kiukaanniemi S, et al. Overweight and obese but not normal weight women with PCOS are at increased risk of Type 2 diabetes mellitus-a prospective, population-based cohort study. *Hum Reprod (Oxf Engl)*. 2017;32(2):423–431. https://doi.org/10.1093/humrep/dew329. [published Online First: Epub Date], with permission.)

HbA1c was less sensitive (60%) and specific (69%) in detecting glucose abnormalities when compared with the OGTT. HbA1c missed four patients with IGT and one patient with IFG on OGTT, while it was elevated in 17 patients with NGT. These results caution against the use of HbA1c as the sole screening tool for dysglycemia in adolescents with PCOS, although it can still be useful because it does not require fasting or a prolonged visit.[49]

Estimations of PCOS in women with diabetes have also been undertaken. Of women who had gestational diabetes, 15%–34% reported irregular menstrual cycles, 18% had hirsutism, and up to 52% had polycystic ovarian morphology on ultrasound evaluation.[50,51] In a study of 38 adult women with T2D, 82% had ultrasound findings of polycystic ovaries and 52% had either clinical hyperandrogenism, menstrual irregularities, or both,[52] while another clinic classified 26.7% of their young women with T2D as having PCOS by chart review.[53]

To summarize, PCOS appears to significantly increase a woman's likelihood of developing T2D, and these patients tend to develop it much earlier in life than women without the disease. Those with obesity and family histories of T2D appear to have a higher risk, while women with PCOS who have a normal BMI exhibit more insulin resistance than women without PCOS. However, their risk for IGT and T2D is less clear.

THE METABOLIC SYNDROME

Women and adolescents with PCOS often have evidence of the metabolic syndrome. Although the term metabolic syndrome generally invokes an understanding of a clustering of diagnoses that increase one's risk for obesity and cardiovascular morbidity, there are several similar definitions that are used throughout the world that adjust the main focus of the syndrome.[54,55] As shown in Table 10.1, the WHO focuses on glucose abnormalities, in addition to the presence of at least two other criteria.[2,54] To meet the International Diabetes Federation's (IDF) diagnosis, a patient must have abdominal adiposity with at least two other criteria.[54] The National Cholesterol Education Program Adult Treatment Panel III (NCEP ATP III) allows for diagnosis if any three criteria are met.[55]

TABLE 10.1

Comparison of the World Health Organization (WHO), International Diabetes Federation (IDF), and National Cholesterol Education Program Adult Treatment Panel III (NCEP ATP III) Definitions of the Metabolic Syndrome

	WHO	IDF	NCEP ATP III
Necessary criteria	Glucose abnormalities + two criteria	Abdominal adiposity + two criteria	Any three criteria
Blood sugar	Fasting glucose >100 mg/dL, 2-h OGTT value >140 mg/dL, abnormal HOMA-IR or hyperinsulinemic euglycemic clamp, or diabetes diagnosis	Fasting glucose >100 mg/dL or type 2 diabetes diagnosis	Fasting glucose >110 mg/dL
Blood pressure	≥140/90 mmHg	≥130 systolic or ≥85 diastolic	>130/85
Triglycerides	>150 mg/dL	≥150 mg/dL	≥150 mg/dL
HDL	<39 mg/dL in women	<40 mg/dL in women	<50 mg/dL in women
Abdominal adiposity	Waist-to-hip ratio >0.85 in women or BMI >30 kg/m²	Waist circumference based on ethnic norms or BMI >30 kg/m²	Waist circumference >88 cm in women
Microalbuminuria	Albumin excretion rate ≥20 μg/min or albumin: creatinine ratio ≥30 mg/g	Not applicable	Not applicable

Abdominal obesity in females with PCOS is not only associated with hypertension, insulin resistance, and T2D, but also elevated triglycerides, elevated LDL, and low HDL.[9] Elevated inflammatory markers have been found in women with PCOS, and the presence of fibrinolytic dysfunction has been suggested by some studies.[9] Together, these risk factors are believed to place women with PCOS at increased risk for future cardiovascular disease (Fig. 10.6).[26]

A recent study examining a large, diverse group of 702 women between 18 and 40 years of age who fit the Rotterdam criteria for PCOS provides evidence that there are also ethnic variations in insulin resistance and the metabolic syndrome.[56] The study included 467 non-Hispanic whites, 98 non-Hispanic blacks, and 128 Hispanic women. There was no difference in obesity as measured by BMI and abdominal circumference among the group. Hispanic women were found to have more hirsutism ($P = .03$), acne ($P < .01$), and higher free androgen index ($P < .01$) secondary to lower SHBG values ($P < .01$). With regard to insulin resistance, Hispanic women were again more affected, with 44.5% having elevated fasting insulin ($P = .03$), higher proinsulin levels ($P = .01$), and over 50% had elevated HOMA-IR levels ($P = .01$). Fasting glucose was ≥100 mg/dL in 14.8% of the Hispanic women, 7.1% of the non-Hispanic blacks, and 6.5% of the non-Hispanic whites ($P = .01$). No difference was found in rates of the metabolic syndrome when study site was controlled for, although

Hispanic and non-Hispanic black patients were more likely to have elevated systolic blood pressure (27.3% and 28.6%, respectively) compared to their non-Hispanic white counterparts (19%, $P = .03$). The non-Hispanic black patients were significantly less likely to experience hypertriglyceridemia (5.1%) compared to the other two groups (28.3% and 30.5%, respectively, $P < .01$).[56]

One thousand eighty-nine women with PCOS and a median age of 28 years were recruited from several clinics in the United States, India, Finland, Norway, and Brazil. Comparisons of the prevalence and components of the metabolic syndrome across different patient populations were made, using the non-Hispanic US white population as a reference group.[57] The researchers found that the non-Hispanic US black women had the highest prevalence of the metabolic syndrome (52%, $P < .001$), and obesity (74%, $P < .001$). This disparity disappeared when adjustment for BMI was considered (odds ratio of the metabolic syndrome dropped from 4.54, $P < .001$ to 1.7, adjusted $P = .18$). Indian and Norwegian women had the highest prevalence of the metabolic syndrome, 38.2% and 41.1%, respectively, which was not attributable to BMI status. Interestingly, the Norwegian women had a much higher prevalence of the metabolic syndrome than their Finnish neighbors (27.7%), who had prevalence rates more similar to the US white women (28.3%).[57]

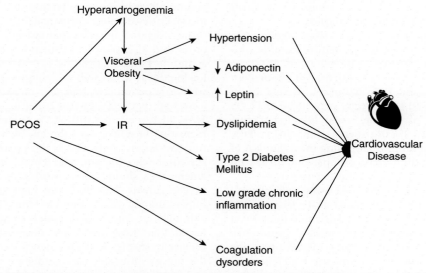

FIG. 10.6 Risk factors associated with PCOS that contribute to cardiovascular disease. *IR*, insulin resistance. (From Orio F, Muscogiuri G, Nese C, et al. Obesity, type 2 diabetes mellitus and cardiovascular disease risk: an uptodate in the management of polycystic ovary syndrome. *Eur J Obstet Gynecol Reprod Biol*. 2016;207:214–219. https://doi.org/10.1016/j.ejogrb.2016.08.026. [published Online First: Epub Date], with permission.)

There was also a significant difference in which the metabolic syndrome abnormalities were predominant in the different groups. In the reference US white women, 47.3% were obese, 20.7% had hypertriglyceridemia, 36.4% were hypertensive, 12% had fasting hyperglycemia, and 41.9% exhibited low HDL levels. The Finnish patients' parameters were not significantly different from the US white patients, and the only difference in the Brazilian patients was a higher percentage of women with low HDL levels (59.2%, $P < .001$). However, non-Hispanic US black women tended to have more obesity (74%, $P < .001$), hypertension (59%, $P < .001$), fasting hyperglycemia (22%, $P < .05$), and low HDL (72%, $P < .001$), with fewer patients exhibiting hypertriglyceridemia (10%, $P < .05$). The Asian Indian patients, while also obese (62.3%, $P < .05$), had more fasting hyperglycemia (28.6%, $P < .001$) and low HDL levels (97.3%, $P < .001$), with fewer of the women meeting criteria for hypertension (16.8%, $P < .001$). The Norwegian women had a combination of hypertension (52.7%, $P < .05$), fasting hyperglycemia (21.7%, $P < .05$), and low HDL levels (59.7%, $P < .001$). This study further highlights the heterogeneity of PCOS among different ethnicities.[57]

Hart et al.[58] used the Western Australia Pregnancy Cohort to investigate the metabolic syndrome in girls carrying the PCOS diagnosis by NIH or Rotterdam Criteria. The metabolic syndrome diagnosis was made by modified IDF, European Group for the Study of Insulin Resistance (EGIR), modified NCEP ATP III, and the WHO criteria. Two hundred forty-four girls between the ages of 14.5 and 17.7 years took part in the study. Nine percent of the teens were obese, 20% were overweight, and the majority of the girls (73%) were over 2 years post-menarche. The diagnosis of the metabolic syndrome ranged from 0.5% (modified NCEP ATP III) to 4.3% (modified IDF) of girls, based on the definition used. Over half of the girls (53.1%) exhibited irregular menstrual cycles, 27.7% had an elevated calculated free testosterone level, and 35.3% had polycystic ovaries on transabdominal ultrasound.

There were significantly more girls who fit Rotterdam and NIH criteria that had waist circumferences over the 90th percentile for age compared to those who did not (45.9% with PCOS via Rotterdam criteria compared to 29.4% who did not $P = .035$, and 61.8% with PCOS via NIH criteria vs. 29% who did not $P = .001$). As would be expected given the above, they also had significantly higher BMIs than the girls who did not have PCOS (24.2 with PCOS via Rotterdam criteria compared to 22.1 $P = .005$, and 25.8 with PCOS via NIH criteria vs. 22.1 $P = .001$). Girls who carried a PCOS diagnosis using either criteria were more likely to fit all of the definitions of the metabolic syndrome.[58]

Median fasting insulin levels were significantly, but not substantially, more elevated in the girls who met PCOS criteria versus those who did not have PCOS (11.1 μU/mL vs. 10.5 μU/mL in Rotterdam patients, $P = .045$, and 11.95 μU/mL vs. 10.3 μU/mL in NIH patients, $P = .014$). A greater percentage of PCOS patients (13.6% of patients using Rotterdam criteria, $P = .007$ and 18.2% of patients using NIH criteria, $P = .007$) were insulin resistant, using the definition of a HOMA-IR calculation over 4, compared to those who did not have PCOS (2.8% and 3.6%, respectively).

Cluster analysis was performed using waist circumference, insulin, HDL, calculated LDL, triglycerides, blood pressure, and glucose to determine the girls at highest risk for developing the metabolic syndrome. Girls with PCOS were more likely to end up in the high-risk cluster. The girls within the high-risk compared to the low-risk cluster had significantly higher waist circumference (85 vs. 71 cm, $P < .001$), higher systolic (117 vs. 108 mm Hg, $P < .001$) and diastolic (63 vs. 59 mm Hg, $P < .001$) blood pressures, lower HDL (1.28 vs. 1.46 mmol/L, $P = .003$), higher triglycerides (1.16 vs. 0.94 mmol/L, $P = .001$), higher CRP (0.58 vs. 0.24 mg/L, $P = .005$), higher insulin levels (13.2 vs. 9.99 μU/mL, $P < .001$), and higher HOMA-IR (2.76 vs. 2.08, $P < .001$). Elevated calculated free testosterone levels correlated with insulin resistance, independent of weight status.[58] Similar findings were demonstrated in an earlier study as well.[26]

To review, several large studies have established that the metabolic syndrome occurs in women and adolescents with PCOS. There also appears to be variation in the components of the metabolic syndrome that preferentially affects different racial and ethnic groups.

PCOS WORKUP

As with all encounters, a thorough history and physical exam are critical to the PCOS workup. Attention should be paid to a past medical history of IUGR or SGA status, premature adrenarche, and/or premature pubarche.[7] Family history may also provide clues, and while there may not be anyone in the family carrying the formal diagnosis of PCOS, one or more women may have struggled with irregular periods, infertility, or hirsutism. Inquiring about family members with obesity, hyperlipidemia, gestational diabetes, or T2D is also important.

Girls with hyperandrogenism who experience early menarche have been found to be at greater risk for

abnormalities in glucose tolerance, and it is imperative to obtain a complete menstrual history.[7] Oligomenorrhea (defined as cycles that last fewer than 20 days or beyond 45 days once a patient is 2 years post-menarche), lack of menarche by 15 years or 2–3 years following thelarche, as well as going longer than 90 days without a period any time after menarche all warrant a workup that includes evaluating for PCOS.[16] Up to 15%–30% of women with PCOS will exhibit monthly menstrual bleeding, even though their cycles are not truly ovulatory, while girls at the opposite end of the spectrum who present with complaints of primary amenorrhea, should also be worked up for PCOS.[2]

The growth chart and vital signs should be carefully examined. PCOS does not typically affect stature, although one study of girls with premature adrenarche found that those who were diagnosed with PCOS achieved a shorter final adult height than the girls who did not go on to develop the disease.[59] Weight, BMI, and waist circumference measurements provide information on the presence, onset, and progression of weight issues. Obesity-related comorbidities, including hypertension, should also be noted.

Acne and hirsutism should be inquired about, particularly because patients may be on acne medications or engage in some form of excess hair removal, making these signs less apparent on exam. When present, the severity of hirsutism should be described according to the Ferriman Gallwey scoring system.[7] Scores of 8 or greater are used in Caucasian and African American populations, although this may be too high in other ethnicities, particularly in Asian females, and cutoffs as low as 3 or 5 have been recommended for them. One should be aware of signs of insulin resistance including acanthosis nigricans and skin tags,[15,16] as well as signs of other potential diagnoses including hypertension, Cushingoid facies, violaceous striae, abnormal growth velocity, café-au-lait macules, clitoromegaly, and thyromegaly. Abrupt loss of menstrual cycles and rapid virilization are concerning clues that necessitate further lab work and imaging to identify androgen-secreting tumors of the ovaries or adrenal glands.[2]

As mentioned earlier, other diseases in which hyperandrogenism and menstrual irregularities may manifest should be ruled out prior to diagnosing PCOS. As such, 17-hydroxyprogesterone should be drawn to screen for nonclassical CAH. Gonadotropins and estradiol are helpful if considering hypogonadotropic hypogonadism and premature ovarian failure, while prolactin, thyroid hormone levels, and ACTH stimulation testing may be obtained if clinically suspecting another cause of the patient's symptoms.[12,16] Prolactin levels are generally normal in females with PCOS, but the value may be slightly elevated in up to 15% of them.[2]

No test is 100% specific for PCOS, but testosterone is the androgen which is most commonly elevated. However, reliable measurement of testosterone can prove difficult, as levels naturally increase with pubertal progression, and adolescent norms have not been established.[16] It is recommended that hyperandrogenemia be diagnosed when testosterone levels are greater than "the adult female normative values according to assays performed by specialty laboratories with well-defined reference intervals" on more than one occasion.[16] Radioimmunoassay and liquid chromatography-mass spectrometry assays are felt to be the most accurate ways to measure total testosterone, while free testosterone is best measured by equilibrium dialysis.[3,16] SHBG levels are critical to interpreting free testosterone levels, and are usually low in girls with PCOS.[3,13,60] SHBG has also been noted to be inversely associated with IR and has been used as a biochemical marker of IR.[23]

DHEA-S is another key marker of hyperandrogenism, and androstenedione may also be elevated.[13,16] Although many patients have been found to have elevated LH to follicle stimulating hormone (FSH) ratios, a lack of standardized cutoff values across different assays, as well as the confounding normalization of LH in obese patients, has made this a less reliable marker than other labs.[13] Lab data are most informative when obtained in the early morning.[7]

Pelvic ultrasonography to evaluate for polycystic ovarian morphology is felt to be of limited value in adolescents. Assessment of the ovaries transabdominally is difficult, particularly in overweight and obese patients, and transvaginal ultrasounds are generally avoided.[7,15,16]

Once a diagnosis of PCOS is established, patients should be screened for associated comorbidities. Given the increased risk for depression and anxiety, referral for therapy is often warranted.[1,11,15] Overweight and obese patients with symptoms of obstructive sleep apnea should obtain a formal sleep study.[15] Alanine aminotransferase (ALT) and aspartate aminotransferase (AST) should be drawn to screen for nonalcoholic fatty liver disease, while a fasting lipid panel is recommended to evaluate for dyslipidemia.[61] As discussed in detail in the insulin resistance, T2D, and the metabolic syndrome sections provided earlier, PCOS predisposes patients to dysglycemia. Women with PCOS more frequently have elevated glucose after meals than when fasting: a sign of insulin resistance in the peripheral tissues.[9] Although easier to complete, a hemoglobin A1c is less effective when screening for dysglycemia in the

PCOS population, and an oral glucose tolerance test should be considered.[15]

THERAPEUTIC APPROACHES

It is generally accepted that lifestyle interventions, including increased physical activity, and dietary counseling should be the first therapies offered to overweight and obese patients with PCOS. Weight loss has been shown to decrease hyperandrogenemia, regulate menstrual cycles, and improve components of the metabolic syndrome.[1,7,15,61]

The Endocrine Society endorses the use of oral contraceptive pills (OCPs) for acne, hirsutism, and anovulation resulting from probable PCOS, and consideration of metformin in girls with impaired glucose tolerance or evidence of the metabolic syndrome.[15] Metformin has been shown in adults to improve ovulatory function and insulin sensitivity mainly through inhibition of hepatic glucose production and increased peripheral tissue insulin sensitivity, as well as decreased ovarian androgen production.[62]

In adolescents, the benefits of metformin are still unclear. Several studies have explored the use of different doses of metformin therapy. Twenty-two Canadian overweight or obese adolescents with PCOS between the ages of 13 and 18 years were provided with healthy lifestyle education and randomized to either metformin 750 mg BID for 3 months or placebo.[63] Although only four of the girls taking the placebo had at least one menstrual cycle, 10 of the 11 girls on metformin achieved this. The patients on metformin had an average drop of 38.3 ng/dL in their total testosterone levels, and a rise of 6.98 mg/dL in their HDL, but the patients on placebo had minimal changes in both. Weight loss and changes in measures of insulin sensitivity and secretion were negligible in both groups. However, gastrointestinal side effects limited adherence to metformin therapy and may have played a part in the investigators' lack of statistically significant findings with regard to insulin sensitivity.

Ibáñez and her group[59] have conducted several studies looking at the use of metformin in girls at risk for or with PCOS. In one study, her team followed 38 girls who were low birth weight and exhibited precocious pubarche secondary to premature adrenarche over a 7-year period. They were randomized to treatment with metformin for the first 4 years (425 mg daily for 2 years, then 850 mg daily for the remaining 2 years) or no medication. The girls who did not receive metformin initially were treated with 850 mg of metformin during year 6. Patients who had received metformin at a younger age were significantly less likely to fit either the Androgen Excess Society or NIH definition of PCOS, reached a taller final adult height, had lower systemic inflammation measured via CRP and neutrophil count, less hirsutism, decreased visceral adiposity, lower BMIs, lower insulin resistance markers, and lower androgen levels. Although the girls treated during year 6 did show improvement in these measures during that time period, it did not last after the medication was discontinued. Based on these results, it has been argued that late childhood may be a critical and promising period for intervention to prevent PCOS progression; much earlier than previously believed.

In another study by Ibáñez and group,[8] 10 nonobese girls with a history of premature pubarche, anovulation, and hyperandrogenism were treated with 1275 mg of metformin daily for 6 months. Ferriman-Gallwey score, testosterone, and DHEA-S all significantly improved with treatment, but rose again within 3 months of discontinuing the medication. Similarly, all girls achieved menstrual regularity within 4 months of starting metformin, but developed oligomenorrhea within 3 months of discontinuation. Although glucose tolerance was normal throughout the study, mean serum insulin improved substantially from 111.2 ± 6.2 mU/L initially to 61.9 ± 8.4 mU/L after 6 months of treatment ($P < .001$), but increased after 3 months off of metformin. SHBG increased significantly, while the lipid panel improved on metformin, with total cholesterol, LDL, and triglycerides significantly lowered, and HDL increasing, although, all showed rebound once the medication was discontinued.

De Leo's group treated 16 obese, anovulatory teenagers (15–18 years old) with PCOS and insulin resistance seen on OGTT with a low carbohydrate, high protein diet, and a higher dose of 1700 mg of metformin daily for 6 months. All of the patients lost weight, normalized their BMI, had biochemical evidence of ovulatory menstrual cycles, and a statistically significant reduction in hyperandrogenemia. In contrast to the previous study, menstrual cycles were still ovulatory 6 months after discontinuation of metformin.[64] Collectively, the aforementioned studies emphasize the importance of insulin resistance in the pathophysiology of PCOS, and imply that improvement in symptoms can be achieved when steps are taken to enhance insulin sensitivity.

In addition to the use of metformin, OCPs are often indicated in the management of PCOS. OCPs promote ovarian quiescence as well as increase SHBG, and in doing so, decrease freely circulating testosterone. As such, patients experience regular periods and improvement in hyperandrogenism. Unfortunately, OCPs do have the unfavorable side effects of increasing LDL, triglycerides, and deep vein thrombosis (DVT), so careful personal and family history with counseling on these risks should be undertaken prior to their prescription.[7]

Studies comparing the use of OCPs to metformin, combination therapy, lifestyle interventions, or placebo have found improvements in different PCOS symptoms and comorbidities. Two small randomized, placebo controlled trials involving patients with a BMI over the 95th percentile, oligomenorrhea, and clinical or biochemical hyperandrogenism from 12 to 18 years of age were undertaken to explore the effects of lifestyle modifications, OCPs, and metformin. In the first trial,[65] 43 patients were randomized to receive either lifestyle interventions, metformin 850 mg BID, placebo, or OCPs for 6 months. The patients on OCPs were the only ones who experienced statistically significant weight loss with improvement in their hyperandrogenism, area under the curve (AUC) insulin, and HDL. However, this was at the expense of elevated LDL and CRP levels. The lifestyle intervention arm also led to a decline in hyperandrogenism. Metformin use decreased triglyceride levels and fasting blood glucose, though there was no improvement in glucose tolerance. The second trial enrolled 36 different patients who received lifestyle interventions and OCPs in combination with 2000 mg/day of metformin or placebo. In this study, there was also some weight loss, but results largely mirrored those seen in the girls on OCPs in the first trial, without benefitting glucose tolerance.[65] A larger study[66] followed 119 Egyptian girls who received either metformin, an OCP, or no therapy for 2 years, and showed improvements in menstrual regularity and hirsutism in the girls receiving therapy, prolonged lowering of serum testosterone in those on OCPs, and improvement in insulin sensitivity measures if taking metformin, but worsening of these measures on OCPs.

Combination therapies using metformin, with flutamide, rosiglitazone, or exenatide, have been trialed in adult women with PCOS.[67-69] Although treatment time has varied from 6 to 12 months, randomized controlled trials have generally shown benefits in weight, ovulation, hyperandrogenism, and insulin resistance. Women on flutamide[67] experienced improvements in visceral and fat mass as well as measures of hyperandrogenemia, although combination therapy with metformin did not appear to enhance the individual drugs' effects. Exenatide is a glucagon like peptide-1 agonist used in T2D to improve insulin secretion, which may secondarily induce weight loss. When Caucasian and African American adult women with PCOS and BMIs over 27 kg/m^2 were treated with exenatide, menstrual, hyperandrogenic, and metabolic indices all improved. Exenatide and metformin together caused mean weight loss of 6 kg, compared to 3.2 kg in the women on exenatide alone, and 1.6 kg in those on metformin. Of the 11 women with glucose intolerance via OGTT, 3/5 on metformin, 1/3 on exenatide, and all three of the women on combination therapy had normalization of the abnormalities by the end of the study.[68] Nonobese Caucasian women of European descent with NGT who were treated with metformin, rosiglitazone, or combination therapy had improved ovulation rates, as well as free and total testosterone levels. Even though the women were not insulin resistant, fasting insulin levels declined significantly in the metformin and combination therapy groups. This study also had the unusual findings of AUC glucose being higher, and decreased glucose tolerance in the women on both metformin and rosiglitazone. Further research is required to elucidate the potential benefits of these drugs in the treatment of PCOS.

Spironolactone is a potassium sparing diuretic that also binds to the androgen receptor, creating anti-androgenic properties.[61] As a result, it works well to improve acne, hirsutism, and hyperandrogenemia in teenagers.[62] As it is teratogenic, spironolactone should be prescribed in conjunction with contraception.[7,61]

Myo-inositol is a compound that is showing promise for improving insulin sensitivity. It is abundant in certain foods, including fruits and whole grains, but can also be produced by the body from glucose. Studies in both normal and overweight patients with PCOS have shown that myo-inositol supplementation causes an androgen lowering effect, and improves glucose tolerance on OGTT when given for 12 weeks or longer. The benefit is hypothesized to derive from myo-inositol's stimulation of inositolphosphoglycans, which are important messengers in the pathway for glucose utilization. Although studies are small, this supplement has the added benefit of not inducing side effects.[70]

Finally, Neurokinin B is believed to regulate LH by acting on the neurokinin 3 receptor and causing GnRH production.[71] Neurokinin 3 receptor antagonists have proven capable of decreasing LH and testosterone levels in women with PCOS, particularly in those who were anovulatory, suggesting that this may become a useful tool in the rather limited arsenal of PCOS therapies.[5,71]

In summary, lifestyle changes, metformin, and the use of OCPs remain the mainstay of PCOS management, particularly in young females. Once diagnosed with type 2 diabetes, glucose and HbA1c should be carefully monitored, as insulin initiation may be necessary. Spironolactone can be a useful adjunct for ameliorating clinical manifestations of hyperandrogenism, although its teratogenic potential requires contraceptive precautions in reproductive aged women. Combination therapies and new therapeutic modalities are constantly being evaluated in hopes of discovering additional and more beneficial regimens for this patient population.

REFERENCES

1. Azziz R, Carmina E, Chen Z, et al. Polycystic ovary syndrome. Nature reviews. *Dis Primers.* 2016;2:16057. https://doi.org/10.1038/nrdp.2016.57. [published Online First: Epub Date].
2. Ovalle F, Azziz R. Insulin resistance, polycystic ovary syndrome, and type 2 diabetes mellitus. *Fertil Steril.* 2002;77(6):1095–1105.
3. Diamanti-Kandarakis E, Dunaif A. Insulin resistance and the polycystic ovary syndrome revisited: an update on mechanisms and implications. *Endocr Rev.* 2012;33(6):981–1030. https://doi.org/10.1210/er.2011-1034. [published Online First: Epub Date].
4. Palmert MR, Gordon CM, Kartashov AI, Legro RS, Emans SJ, Dunaif A. Screening for abnormal glucose tolerance in adolescents with polycystic ovary syndrome. *J Clin Endocrinol Metab.* 2002;87(3):1017–1023. https://doi.org/10.1210/jcem.87.3.8305. [published Online First: Epub Date].
5. Baldauff NH, Witchel SF. Polycystic ovary syndrome in adolescent girls. *Curr Opin Endocrinol Diabetes Obes.* 2017;24(1):56–66. https://doi.org/10.1097/MED.0000000000000309. [published Online First: Epub Date].
6. Harwood K, Vuguin P, DiMartino-Nardi J. Current approaches to the diagnosis and treatment of polycystic ovarian syndrome in youth. *Horm Res.* 2007;68(5):209–217. https://doi.org/10.1159/000101538. [published Online First: Epub Date].
7. Ibanez L, Ong KK, Lopez-Bermejo A, Dunger DB, de Zegher F. Hyperinsulinaemic androgen excess in adolescent girls. *Nat Rev Endocrinol.* 2014;10(8):499–508. https://doi.org/10.1038/nrendo.2014.58. [published Online First: Epub Date].
8. Ibanez L, Valls C, Potau N, Marcos MV, de Zegher F. Sensitization to insulin in adolescent girls to normalize hirsutism, hyperandrogenism, oligomenorrhea, dyslipidemia, and hyperinsulinism after precocious pubarche. *J Clin Endocrinol Metab.* 2000;85(10):3526–3530. https://doi.org/10.1210/jcem.85.10.6908. [published Online First: Epub Date].
9. Orio F, Muscogiuri G, Nese C, et al. Obesity, type 2 diabetes mellitus and cardiovascular disease risk: an uptodate in the management of polycystic ovary syndrome. *Eur J Obstet Gynecol Reprod Biol.* 2016;207:214–219. https://doi.org/10.1016/j.ejogrb.2016.08.026. [published Online First: Epub Date].

10. Franks S. Polycystic ovary syndrome in adolescents. *Int J Obes (Lond)*. 2008;32(7):1035–1041. https://doi.org/10.1038/ijo.2008.61. [published Online First: Epub Date].
11. Anderson AD, Solorzano CM, McCartney CR. Childhood obesity and its impact on the development of adolescent PCOS. *Semin. Reprod Med.* 2014;32(3):202–213. https://doi.org/10.1055/s-0034-1371092. [published Online First: Epub Date].
12. Revised 2003 consensus on diagnostic criteria and long-term health risks related to polycystic ovary syndrome (PCOS). *Hum Reprod (Oxf Engl)*. 2004;19(1):41–47.
13. Azziz R, Carmina E, Dewailly D, et al. The Androgen Excess and PCOS Society criteria for the polycystic ovary syndrome: the complete task force report. *Fertil Steril.* 2009;91(2):456–488. https://doi.org/10.1016/j.fertnstert.2008.06.035. [published Online First: Epub Date].
14. NIH. *Executive Summary. Evidence-Based Methodology Workshop on Polycystic Ovary Syndrome.* Bethesda, Maryland: National Institutes of Health; 2012:1–14.
15. Legro RS, Arslanian SA, Ehrmann DA, et al. Diagnosis and treatment of polycystic ovary syndrome: an endocrine society clinical practice guideline. *J Clin Endocrinol Metab.* 2013;98(12):4565–4592. https://doi.org/10.1210/jc.2013-2350. [published Online First: Epub Date].
16. Witchel SF, Oberfield S, Rosenfield RL, et al. *The Diagnosis of Polycystic Ovary Syndrome during Adolescence.* Horm Res Paediatr; 2015. https://doi.org/10.1159/000375530. [published Online First: Epub Date].
17. Kyritsi EM, Dimitriadis GK, Kyrou I, Kaltsas G, Randeva HS. PCOS remains a diagnosis of exclusion: a concise review of key endocrinopathies to exclude. *Clin Endocrinol.* 2017;86(1):1–6. https://doi.org/10.1111/cen.13245. [published Online First: Epub Date].
18. Consensus Development Conference on Insulin Resistance. American diabetes association. *Diabetes Care 1998.* November 5–6, 1997;21(2):310–314.
19. Matthews DR, Hosker JP, Rudenski AS, Naylor BA, Treacher DF, Turner RC. Homeostasis model assessment: insulin resistance and beta-cell function from fasting plasma glucose and insulin concentrations in man. *Diabetologia.* 1985;28(7):412–419.
20. Lim SS, Davies MJ, Norman RJ, Moran LJ. Overweight, obesity and central obesity in women with polycystic ovary syndrome: a systematic review and meta-analysis. *Hum Reprod Update.* 2012;18(6):618–637. https://doi.org/10.1093/humupd/dms030. [published Online First: Epub Date].
21. Christensen SB, Black MH, Smith N, et al. Prevalence of polycystic ovary syndrome in adolescents. *Fertil Steril.* 2013;100(2):470–477. https://doi.org/10.1016/j.fertnstert.2013.04.001. [published Online First: Epub Date].
22. Dunaif A, Segal KR, Futterweit W, Dobrjansky A. Profound peripheral insulin resistance, independent of obesity, in polycystic ovary syndrome. *Diabetes.* 1989;38(9):1165–1174.
23. Cassar S, Misso ML, Hopkins WG, Shaw CS, Teede HJ, Stepto NK. Insulin resistance in polycystic ovary syndrome: a systematic review and meta-analysis of euglycaemic-hyperinsulinaemic clamp studies. *Hum Reprod (Oxf Engl)*. 2016;31(11):2619–2631. https://doi.org/10.1093/humrep/dew243. [published Online First: Epub Date].
24. Legro RS, Finegood D, Dunaif A. A fasting glucose to insulin ratio is a useful measure of insulin sensitivity in women with polycystic ovary syndrome. *J Clin Endocrinol Metab.* 1998;83(8):2694–2698. https://doi.org/10.1210/jcem.83.8.5054. [published Online First: Epub Date].
25. Carmina E, Koyama T, Chang L, Stanczyk FZ, Lobo RA. Does ethnicity influence the prevalence of adrenal hyperandrogenism and insulin resistance in polycystic ovary syndrome? *Am J Obstet Gynecol.* 1992;167(6):1807–1812.
26. Fruzzetti F, Perini D, Lazzarini V, Parrini D, Genazzani AR. Adolescent girls with polycystic ovary syndrome showing different phenotypes have a different metabolic profile associated with increasing androgen levels. *Fertil Steril.* 2009;92(2):626–634. https://doi.org/10.1016/j.fertnstert.2008.06.004. [published Online First: Epub Date].
27. Lewy VD, Danadian K, Witchel SF, Arslanian S. Early metabolic abnormalities in adolescent girls with polycystic ovarian syndrome. *J Pediatr.* 2001;138(1):38–44. https://doi.org/10.1067/mpd.2001.109603. [published Online First: Epub Date].
28. Apter D, Butzow T, Laughlin GA, Yen SS. Metabolic features of polycystic ovary syndrome are found in adolescent girls with hyperandrogenism. *J Clin Endocrinol Metab.* 1995;80(10):2966–2973. https://doi.org/10.1210/jcem.80.10.7559882. [published Online First: Epub Date].
29. Soto N, Bazaes RA, Pena V, et al. Insulin sensitivity and secretion are related to catch-up growth in small-for-gestational-age infants at age 1 year: results from a prospective cohort. *J Clin Endocrinol Metab.* 2003;88(8):3645–3650. https://doi.org/10.1210/jc.2002-030031. [published Online First: Epub Date].
30. Veening MA, Van Weissenbruch MM, Delemarre-Van De Waal HA. Glucose tolerance, insulin sensitivity, and insulin secretion in children born small for gestational age. *J Clin Endocrinol Metab.* 2002;87(10):4657–4661. https://doi.org/10.1210/jc.2001-011940. [published Online First: Epub Date].
31. McCartney CR, Prendergast KA, Chhabra S, et al. The association of obesity and hyperandrogenemia during the pubertal transition in girls: obesity as a potential factor in the genesis of postpubertal hyperandrogenism. *J Clin Endocrinol Metab.* 2006;91(5):1714–1722. https://doi.org/10.1210/jc.2005-1852. [published Online First: Epub Date].
32. Davies MJ, March WA, Willson KJ, Giles LC, Moore VM. Birthweight and thinness at birth independently predict symptoms of polycystic ovary syndrome in adulthood. *Hum Reprod (Oxf Engl)*. 2012;27(5):1475–1480. https://doi.org/10.1093/humrep/des027. [published Online First: Epub Date].

33. Cresswell JL, Barker DJ, Osmond C, Egger P, Phillips DI, Fraser RB. Fetal growth, length of gestation, and polycystic ovaries in adult life. *Lancet.* 1997;350(9085):1131–1135.

34. Venkatesan AM, Dunaif A, Corbould A. Insulin resistance in polycystic ovary syndrome: progress and paradoxes. *Recent Prog Horm Res.* 2001;56:295–308.

35. Ehrmann DA, Sturis J, Byrne MM, Karrison T, Rosenfield RL, Polonsky KS. Insulin secretory defects in polycystic ovary syndrome. Relationship to insulin sensitivity and family history of non-insulin-dependent diabetes mellitus. *J Clin Investig.* 1995;96(1):520–527. https://doi.org/10.1172/JCI118064. [published Online First: Epub Date].

36. Dunaif A, Segal KR, Shelley DR, Green G, Dobrjansky A, Licholai T. Evidence for distinctive and intrinsic defects in insulin action in polycystic ovary syndrome. *Diabetes.* 1992;41(10):1257–1266.

37. Dunaif A, Xia J, Book CB, Schenker E, Tang Z. Excessive insulin receptor serine phosphorylation in cultured fibroblasts and in skeletal muscle. A potential mechanism for insulin resistance in the polycystic ovary syndrome. *J Clin Investig.* 1995;96(2):801–810. https://doi.org/10.1172/JCI118126. [published Online First: Epub Date].

38. Ciaraldi TP, el-Roeiy A, Madar Z, Reichart D, Olefsky JM, Yen SS. Cellular mechanisms of insulin resistance in polycystic ovarian syndrome. *J Clin Endocrinol Metab.* 1992;75(2):577–583. https://doi.org/10.1210/jcem.75.2.1322430. [published Online First: Epub Date].

39. Ciaraldi TP, Morales AJ, Hickman MG, Odom-Ford R, Olefsky JM, Yen SS. Cellular insulin resistance in adipocytes from obese polycystic ovary syndrome subjects involves adenosine modulation of insulin sensitivity. *J Clin Endocrinol Metab.* 1997;82(5):1421–1425. https://doi.org/10.1210/jcem.82.5.3961. [published Online First: Epub Date].

40. Griffin ME, Marcucci MJ, Cline GW, et al. Free fatty acid-induced insulin resistance is associated with activation of protein kinase C theta and alterations in the insulin signaling cascade. *Diabetes.* 1999;48(6):1270–1274.

41. Dresner A, Laurent D, Marcucci M, et al. Effects of free fatty acids on glucose transport and IRS-1-associated phosphatidylinositol 3-kinase activity. *J Clin Investig.* 1999;103(2):253–259. https://doi.org/10.1172/JCI5001. [published Online First: Epub Date].

42. Bergman RN, Mittelman SD. Central role of the adipocyte in insulin resistance. *J Basic Clin Physiol Pharmacol.* 1998;9(2–4):205–221.

43. Legro RS, Kunselman AR, Dodson WC, Dunaif A. Prevalence and predictors of risk for type 2 diabetes mellitus and impaired glucose tolerance in polycystic ovary syndrome: a prospective, controlled study in 254 affected women. *J Clin Endocrinol Metab.* 1999;84(1):165–169. https://doi.org/10.1210/jcem.84.1.5393. [published Online First: Epub Date].

44. Ehrmann DA, Barnes RB, Rosenfield RL, Cavaghan MK, Imperial J. Prevalence of impaired glucose tolerance and diabetes in women with polycystic ovary syndrome. *Diabetes Care.* 1999;22(1):141–146.

45. Velija-Asimi Z, Burekovic A, Dujic T, Dizdarevic-Bostandzic A, Semiz S. Incidence of prediabetes and risk of developing cardiovascular disease in women with polycystic ovary syndrome. *Bosnian J Basic Med Sci.* 2016;16(4):298–306. https://doi.org/10.17305/bjbms.2016.1428. [published Online First: Epub Date].

46. Ollila ME, West S, Keinanen-Kiukaanniemi S, et al. Overweight and obese but not normal weight women with PCOS are at increased risk of Type 2 diabetes mellitus-a prospective, population-based cohort study. *Hum Reprod (Oxf Engl).* 2017;32(2):423–431. https://doi.org/10.1093/humrep/dew329. [published Online First: Epub Date].

47. Dahlgren E, Johansson S, Lindstedt G, et al. Women with polycystic ovary syndrome wedge resected in 1956 to 1965: a long-term follow-up focusing on natural history and circulating hormones. *Fertil Steril.* 1992;57(3):505–513.

48. Coles N, Bremer K, Kives S, Zhao X, Hamilton J. Utility of the oral glucose tolerance test to assess glucose abnormalities in adolescents with polycystic ovary syndrome. *J Pediatr Adolesc Gynecol.* 2016;29(1):48–52. https://doi.org/10.1016/j.jpag.2015.06.004. [published Online First: Epub Date].

49. Gooding HC, Milliren C, St Paul M, Mansfield MJ, DiVasta A. Diagnosing dysglycemia in adolescents with polycystic ovary syndrome. *J Adolesc Health.* 2014;55(1):79–84. https://doi.org/10.1016/j.jadohealth.2013.12.020. [published Online First: Epub Date].

50. Holte J, Gennarelli G, Wide L, Lithell H, Berne C. High prevalence of polycystic ovaries and associated clinical, endocrine, and metabolic features in women with previous gestational diabetes mellitus. *J Clin Endocrinol Metab.* 1998;83(4):1143–1150. https://doi.org/10.1210/jcem.83.4.4707. [published Online First: Epub Date].

51. Kousta E, Cela E, Lawrence N, et al. The prevalence of polycystic ovaries in women with a history of gestational diabetes. *Clin Endocrinol.* 2000;53(4):501–507.

52. Conn JJ, Jacobs HS, Conway GS. The prevalence of polycystic ovaries in women with type 2 diabetes mellitus. *Clin Endocrinol.* 2000;52(1):81–86.

53. Peppard HR, Marfori J, Iuorno MJ, Nestler JE. Prevalence of polycystic ovary syndrome among premenopausal women with type 2 diabetes. *Diabetes Care.* 2001;24(6):1050–1052.

54. Huang PL. A comprehensive definition for metabolic syndrome. *Dis Model Mech.* 2009;2(5–6):231–237. https://doi.org/10.1242/dmm.001180. [published Online First: Epub Date].

55. Parikh RM, Mohan V. Changing definitions of metabolic syndrome. *Indian J Endocrinol Metab.* 2012;16(1):7–12. https://doi.org/10.4103/2230-8210.91175. [published Online First: Epub Date].

56. Engmann L, Jin S, Sun F, et al. Racial and ethnic differences in the polycystic ovary syndrome metabolic phenotype. *Am J Obstet Gynecol.* 2017. https://doi.org/10.1016/j.ajog.2017.01.003. [published Online First: Epub Date].

57. Chan JL, Kar S, Vanky E, et al. Racial and ethnic differences in the prevalence of metabolic syndrome and its components of metabolic syndrome in women with polycystic ovary syndrome: a regional cross-sectional study. *Am J Obstet Gynecol.* 2017. https://doi.org/10.1016/j.ajog.2017.04.007. [published Online First: Epub Date].

58. Hart R, Doherty DA, Mori T, et al. Extent of metabolic risk in adolescent girls with features of polycystic ovary syndrome. *Fertil Steril.* 2011;95(7):2347–2353. https://doi.org/10.1016/j.fertnstert.2011.03.001. [published Online First: Epub Date].

59. Ibanez L, Lopez-Bermejo A, Diaz M, Marcos MV, de Zegher F. Early metformin therapy (age 8-12 years) in girls with precocious pubarche to reduce hirsutism, androgen excess, and oligomenorrhea in adolescence. *J Clin Endocrinol Metab.* 2011;96(8):E1262–E1267. https://doi.org/10.1210/jc.2011-0555. [published Online First: Epub Date].

60. Driscoll DA. Polycystic ovary syndrome in adolescence. *Ann N Y Acad Sci.* 2003;997:49–55.

61. Hecht Baldauff N, Arslanian S. Optimal management of polycystic ovary syndrome in adolescence. *Arch Dis Childhood.* 2015;100(11):1076–1083. https://doi.org/10.1136/archdischild-2014-306471. [published Online First: Epub Date].

62. Ganie MA, Khurana ML, Eunice M, et al. Comparison of efficacy of spironolactone with metformin in the management of polycystic ovary syndrome: an open-labeled study. *J Clin Endocrinol Metab.* 2004;89(6):2756–2762. https://doi.org/10.1210/jc.2003-031780. [published Online First: Epub Date].

63. Bridger T, MacDonald S, Baltzer F, Rodd C. Randomized placebo-controlled trial of metformin for adolescents with polycystic ovary syndrome. *Arch Pediatr Adolesc Med.* 2006;160(3):241–246. https://doi.org/10.1001/archpedi.160.3.241. [published Online First: Epub Date].

64. De Leo V, Musacchio MC, Morgante G, Piomboni P, Petraglia F. Metformin treatment is effective in obese teenage girls with PCOS. *Hum Reprod (Oxf Engl).* 2006;21(9):2252–2256. https://doi.org/10.1093/humrep/del185. [published Online First: Epub Date].

65. Hoeger K, Davidson K, Kochman L, Cherry T, Kopin L, Guzick DS. The impact of metformin, oral contraceptives, and lifestyle modification on polycystic ovary syndrome in obese adolescent women in two randomized, placebo-controlled clinical trials. *J Clin Endocrinol Metab.* 2008;93(11):4299–4306. https://doi.org/10.1210/jc.2008-0461. [published Online First: Epub Date].

66. El Maghraby HA, Nafee T, Guiziry D, Elnashar A. Randomized controlled trial of the effects of metformin versus combined oral contraceptives in adolescent PCOS women through a 24month follow up period. *Middle East Fertil Soc J.* 2015;20(3):131–137. https://doi.org/10.1016/j.mefs.2014.10.003. [published Online First: Epub Date].

67. Gambineri A, Patton L, Vaccina A, et al. Treatment with flutamide, metformin, and their combination added to a hypocaloric diet in overweight-obese women with polycystic ovary syndrome: a randomized, 12-month, placebo-controlled study. *J Clin Endocrinol Metab.* 2006;91(10):3970–3980. https://doi.org/10.1210/jc.2005-2250. [published Online First: Epub Date].

68. Elkind-Hirsch K, Marrioneaux O, Bhushan M, Vernor D, Bhushan R. Comparison of single and combined treatment with exenatide and metformin on menstrual cyclicity in overweight women with polycystic ovary syndrome. *J Clin Endocrinol Metab.* 2008;93(7):2670–2678. https://doi.org/10.1210/jc.2008-0115. [published Online First: Epub Date].

69. Baillargeon JP, Jakubowicz DJ, Iuorno MJ, Jakubowicz S, Nestler JE. Effects of metformin and rosiglitazone, alone and in combination, in nonobese women with polycystic ovary syndrome and normal indices of insulin sensitivity. *Fertil Steril.* 2004;82(4):893–902. https://doi.org/10.1016/j.fertnstert.2004.02.127. [published Online First: Epub Date].

70. Mansour A, Hosseini S, Larijani B, Mohajeri-Tehrani MR. Nutrients as novel therapeutic approaches for metabolic disturbances in polycystic ovary syndrome. *EXCLI J.* 2016;15:551–564. https://doi.org/10.17179/excli2016-422. [published Online First: Epub Date].

71. George JT, Kakkar R, Marshall J, et al. Neurokinin B receptor antagonism in women with polycystic ovary syndrome: a randomized, placebo-controlled trial. *J Clin Endocrinol Metab.* 2016;101(11):4313–4321. https://doi.org/10.1210/jc.2016-1202. [published Online First: Epub Date].

CHAPTER 11

Pediatric Nonalcoholic Fatty Liver Disease (NAFLD) and Type 2 Diabetes: Pathophysiologic Links and Potential Implications

ALFONSO GALDERISI, MD • MARIANGELA MARTINO, MD • NICOLA SANTORO, MD, PHD

EPIDEMIOLOGY OF PEDIATRIC FATTY LIVER DISEASE

Nonalcoholic fatty liver disease (NAFLD) is a significant global health burden in children, adolescents, and adults with progressive rise in prevalence over the last decades.[1] With the increasing trend in obesity, NAFLD has now become the most common cause of chronic liver disease in children and adolescents, with a prevalence ranging from 3% to 10% in the general pediatric population increasing to up to 70% in obese population.[2]

This condition includes a broad spectrum of liver diseases ranging from simple steatosis to nonalcoholic steatohepatitis with further progression to fibrosis or cirrhosis.[2]

The prevalence of hepatic steatosis varies among different ethnic groups.[3] Hispanics exhibit the highest prevalence of disease, followed by Caucasians and African-Americans.[4] African-Americans instead seem to be protected from hepatic damage even in the presence of a high degree of hepatic fat accumulation and insulin resistance.[5,6]

In addition, gender represents a critical risk factor for the development of NAFLD. In fact, NAFLD is more common in boys than in girls with a male-to-female ratio of 2:1. This has been explained by the liver-protective role of estrogens, as well as by the potentially negative role of androgens in aggravating nonalcoholic steatohepatitis (NASH). The beneficial effects of estrogens on liver could be mediated by the beneficial effect on insulin action.[6]

NAFLD is an independent risk factor for impaired glucose tolerance, with an inverse relationship between hepatic fat content and insulin sensitivity.[7] Nearly 30% of children with NAFLD have abnormal glucose metabolism, with 6.5% developing type 2 diabetes (T2D); whereas, children with T2D have a risk three times greater of developing NASH than those without T2D.[8]

PATHOPHYSIOLOGY OF NAFLD

The liver represents a key hub for both lipid and glucose metabolism, whose interplay underpins the epidemiological overlap between NAFLD and impairment of glucose tolerance[9,10] (Fig. 11.1). NAFLD is associated with hepatic and peripheral insulin resistance, resulting in an insufficient suppression of hepatic gluconeogenesis, decreased glycogen synthesis, and increased lipid accumulation.[9] Although it is clear that β-cell dysfunction is the main factor responsible for the progression to hyperglycemia, insulin resistance precedes β-cell dysfunction and reversibility of insulin resistance delays and prevents the development of diabetes.[11]

Multiple pathways contribute to the development and progression of insulin resistance and consequently to the impairment of β-cell function, including the following:
- Increased lipid availability is strongly associated with both β-cell dysfunction and insulin resistance, that feature type 2 diabetes. Protein kinase C (PKC) family mediates the effects of fat overload, as they are lipid-dependent kinases with wide-ranging roles in signal transduction, including the positive and negative modulation of insulin action[9];
- the inflammatory pathways (reactive oxygen species (ROS), NF-kβ, TNFα, RANKL, caspase 1, IL-1β, IL-6, IL-18)[12];
- the abnormal levels of adipocytokines[13];
- the abnormal fat distribution in obese (increase of visceral and subcutaneous depots and presence of ectopic fat).[14]

Pediatric Type II Diabetes. https://doi.org/10.1016/B978-0-323-55138-0.00011-5.

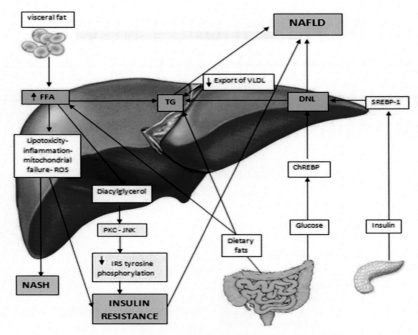

FIG. 11.1 Pathogenic mechanisms leading to NAFLD and insulin resistance.

The increase of lipid flux from gut and adipose tissue to liver is a key feature of NAFLD.[15,16]

Studies of hepatic vein catheterization and isotopic dilution provide evidence that the amount of portal fatty acids derived from visceral fat is increased in obese individuals as compared with lean. This means that an increased fat accumulation in the visceral fat, within an insulin resistance milieu, is responsible for a massive flux of free fatty acids (FFA) to the liver, thus contributing to intrahepatic fat accumulation.[12] Along with the increased flux of FFA from adipose tissue to the liver, also hepatic de novo lipogenesis (DNL), that is the conversion of carbohydrates into fat, strongly contributes to intrahepatic fat accumulation. In fact, seminal studies from Elizabeth Parks have been able to dissect the contribution of dietary fat, adipose tissue lipolysis, and DNL to the intrahepatic fat accumulation. Those studies have shown that about 60% of the fat present in the liver derives from adipose tissue lipolysis, 15% from the diet through the deposition of the fat present in the chylomicron remnants and that DNL contribute for about 25% intrahepatic fat.[17,18]

DNL is increased by Sterol Regulatory Element Binding-Protein 1c (SREBP-1c) and Carbohydrate Response Element Binding-Protein (ChREBP), two transcription factors involved in the regulation of glucose metabolism and lipogenesis. SREBP-1c can bind sterol regulatory elements (SRE) and activate the glucokinase (GK) promoter. SREBP-1c is also able to induce lipogenic genes by its capacity to bind SREs genes on their promoters. SREBP-1c itself is rapidly induced by insulin in primary cultures of hepatocytes.[19] On the other hand, ChREBP is known to recognize E box sequences in the promoters of genes involved in glucose metabolism and it is predominantly expressed in liver, kidney, and adipose tissue. ChREBP is regulated in a reciprocal manner by glucose and cAMP.[19]

All the genetic and environmental factors that interact with the above-mentioned mechanisms are expected to contribute to the individual risk for NAFLD.

Evidence for genetic determinants of NAFLD derive from genome wide association study (GWAS) conducted in both pediatric and adult cohorts.[20] Variants in three genes have been consistently linked to NAFLD in both children and adults: the Patatin-like phospholipase domain-containing protein 3 (PNPLA3), or adiponutrin (ADPN),[21] the Glucokinase Regulatory Protein (GCKR), and the Transmembrane 6 Superfamily Member 2 (TM6SF2).[22]

PNPLA3 encodes for a transmembrane protein expressed in both liver and adipose tissue, the risky variant associated with NAFLD (I148M, rs738409) is featured by a loss of function in its catabolic activity in tryacilglycerol.[23] Although PNPLA3 has not been linked to changes in lipid profile, the polymorphism of GCKR, associated with NAFLD, has been associated to an increase in triglycerides as well as hyperglycemia.[24,25] The gene encodes for a GK regulatory protein whose variation results in an increase of active GK and, consequently, of glucose-6-phosphate that ends up in an increase of DNL.[26] TM6SF2 rs58542926 variant was associated with high hepatic triglycerides content and elevated liver enzymes serum levels,[22] and an impairment of very low density lipoprotein (VLDL) secretion. The three variants of these genes, *PNPLA3*rs738409, *GCKR* rs1260326, and *TM6SF2* rs58542926, have an additive effect on hepatic fat deposition.[27,28]

Beside the individual genetic risk for impaired hepatic lipid processing and storage, dietary is another key influencer for the development of fatty liver in children, as well as in adults.

The consumption of sugar-sweetened beverages in children largely exceed current recommendation,[29] and has been claimed to be involved in future development of diabetes, cardiovascular disease, and fatty liver accumulation. Beverages, but also foods, are often sweetened with sucrose or high-fructose corn syrup, whose ultimate catabolic products are glucose and fructose. Although glucose determinates a pronounced insulin secretion, fructose is not an insulin secretagogue, and increases the expression of enzymes involved in fatty acids' synthesis. Fructose is known to stimulate de novo hepatic lipogenesis by inducing the Srebp-1c and Chrebp-β transcription factors.[30] A pediatric trial has demonstrated that a short-term fructose restriction could be able to reduce liver and visceral fat and DNL with respect to the baseline values, supporting a role for this monosaccharides in the pathogenesis of fatty liver.[31]

Additionally, fructose intake has been demonstrated to influence gut microbiota, both of them affecting the bacterial composition of the intestinal microbiota and impairing the intestinal permeability to bacteria and their endotoxins.[32-34]

Intestinal microbiota, after diet and genome, can be considered the third major player in determining the development of NAFLD, resulting from the interplay of all the three components.

The disruption of gut microbiota, also referred as dysbiosis, has been linked to NAFLD.[35]

Indeed, the microbiota exerts its effect both at luminal level and on the gut mucosal with at least five known mechanisms[36]:

1. short chain fatty acids (SCFA) are a major product of intestinal bacteria, and their disrupted synthesis due to dysbiosis or dietary imbalance contributes to the development of NAFLD. SCFAs exert their action by stimulating luminal G-protein-coupled receptors, and causing the release of intestinal peptides, such as peptide YY (PYY) and glucagon-like peptide 1 (GLP-1), involved in the appetite and insulin secretion. Additionally SCFAs influence directly liver metabolism, increasing hepatic FFA accumulation via decreased β-oxidation.[36] Obese youths show a different gut flora composition than lean subjects, and, on top of the above-mentioned potential mechanisms, their gut microbiota have a higher capability to oxidize carbohydrate that results in an increased amount of SCFA in this group.[37]
2. inhibits the secretion of fasting induced adipose factor (FIAF, also known as angiopoietin-related protein4) which regulates the endothelial lipoprotein lipase (LPL), with the ultimate effect of increasing triglycerides content in circulating chylomicrons and VLDL and their storage in adipocytes and liver.[38]
3. enhanced lipopolysaccharide (LPS) production with the consequent activation of proinflammatory pathways that sustain NAFLD progression.[36]
4. increased endogenous alcohol production that damages tight junctions allowing endotoxins and ethanol to have direct effects on the liver.[36]
5. increased metabolism of dietary phosphatidylcholine (PDC) in gut with a reduced availability of this component for VLDL synthesis and the consequent enhanced accumulation of hepatic triglycerides.[39]

CLINICAL DIAGNOSIS OF NAFLD

NAFLD is a term referring to a wide spectrum of disease. It indicates fatty infiltration in the absence of significant alcohol, genetic diseases, or medications that cause steatosis. Fatty infiltration is typically defined as fat exceeds 5% of the liver by imaging, direct quantification, or histologic estimations.[6] Nonalcoholic fatty liver (NAFL) refers to steatosis without specific changes to suggest steatohepatitis, with or without fibrosis. NASH is a hepatic steatosis with inflammation, with or without ballooning injury to hepatocytes and fibrosis. Therefore, the disease can progress from simple steatosis to fibrosis and cirrhosis.

NAFLD is asymptomatic and for this reason the screening of at-risk individuals is important. According to the current expert guidelines, the screening for NAFLD in pediatrics should be considered between ages 9 and 11 years for all obese children

(BMI ≥ 95th percentile) and mostly for overweight children (BMI ≥ 85th and ≤ 94th percentile) with additional risk factors (central adiposity, insulin resistance, prediabetes or diabetes, dyslipidemia, sleep apnea, or family history of NAFLD/NASH).[40] Earlier screening can be considered in younger patients with risk factors such as severe obesity, family history of NAFLD/NASH, or hypopituitarism.[40] It should be considered to screen the siblings and parents of children with NAFLD if they have known risk factors for it (obesity, Hispanic ethnicity, insulin resistance, prediabetes, diabetes, dyslipidemia).[40]

Plasma measure of alanine-aminotransferase (ALT) is the current screening test for NAFLD. Sex-specific upper limit of normal in children for ALT is 22 U/L for girls and 26 U/L for boys.[40] When the initial screening test is normal, it is advisable to repeat the measurement every 2–3 years if risk factors remain unchanged. These tests should be repeated sooner if clinical risk factors of NAFLD increase in number or severity.[40] Persistently elevated ALT (>3 months) more than twice the upper limit of normal should be evaluated for NAFLD or other causes of chronic hepatitis. When evaluating a child suspected to have NAFLD, alternative etiologies for elevated ALT should be excluded. In fact, without liver biopsy, the diagnosis of NAFLD remains a diagnosis of exclusion.[41] NASH is more common in children with ALT ≥ 80 U/L and the increase of AST/ALT ratio is a sign of advanced fibrosis and cirrhosis.[20]

Clinically available routine ultrasound is not recommended as a screening test for NAFLD in children due to inadequate sensitivity and specificity but it is useful to exclude hepatic masses, cysts, or gallbladder pathology.[40] When available, magnetic resonance imaging and spectroscopy (MRI and MRS) are highly accurate for estimating steatosis while transient elastography and magnetic resonance elastography are the best available assessments of hepatic fibrosis.[42,43] Magnetic resonance elastography (MRE) has been used for clinical evaluation of liver fibrosis for nearly a decade since its first clinical application in 2007.[44] MRE has proven to be an accurate, reproducible, and reliable noninvasive technique for detection and staging of liver fibrosis caused by many different chronic liver diseases. MRE, different from other elastography techniques provides a stiffness map (elastogram) that displays stiffnesses of tissues in large areas across the abdomen. This provides an opportunity for the assessment of stiffness distribution not only within the liver but also other abdominal organs.[45]

Liver biopsy is the current gold standard for the assessment of NAFLD in children and is useful to discriminate between NAFLD and alternative and/or concurrent diagnoses.[46] To assess progression of disease (particularly fibrosis) and to guide treatment is reasonable to consider to repeat liver biopsy 2–3 years after the first liver biopsy, especially in patients with new or ongoing risk factors, such as type 2 diabetes mellitus, NASH, or fibrosis at diagnosis.[40]

NAFLD and Glucose Metabolism

Children with NAFLD should be screened for dyslipidemia and diabetes (at diagnosis and annually, or sooner if clinical suspicion arises) using either a fasting serum glucose level or an HbA1c level (Fig. 11.2). A glucose tolerance test may be useful if the fasting glucose or HbA1c is in the prediabetic range.[40] The risk of T2DM (prediabetes) is defined as an HbA1c of 5.7%–6.4%, impaired fasting glucose level (5.55–6.94 mmol/L or ≥ 100 mg/dL) and/or impaired glucose tolerance (IGT) (7.77–11.04 mmol/L or 140–199 mg/dL at 2h during the standardized 75 g OGTT).[9] The diagnostic criteria for diabetes mellitus from American Diabetes Association are as follows:

- Symptoms of diabetes mellitus (polyuria, polydipsia, and unexplained weight loss with glucosuria and ketonuria) plus random or casual plasma glucose ≥ 200 mg/dL (≥ 11.1 mmol/L);
- Fasting (at least 8h) plasma glucose ≥ 126 mg/dL (≥ 7.0 mmol/L);
- 2h plasma glucose during the OGTT ≥ 200 mg/dL (≥ 11.1 mmol/L);
- Hemoglobin A1c ≥ 6.5%.

Please see Chapters 4 and 5 for additional information on the diagnosis of prediabetes and T2D.

PATHOPHYSIOLOGIC LINK BETWEEN NAFLD AND TYPE 2 DIABETES

Type 2 diabetes results from an imbalance between insulin sensitivity and secretion. Several conditions can influence these two factors (e.g., genetics, diet, physical activity, etc.). The first step in the development of type 2 diabetes in youth is the onset of obesity and its consequences. In particular, obesity is accompanied by an abnormal distribution of lipid partitioning with the excess lipids being diverted from adipose tissue into other organs (such as skeletal muscle and liver).[47] The ectopic fat distribution causes intracellular modifications, which in turn leads to an insulin resistance. A previous study has shown that obese youth with impaired glucose tolerance show a higher intramyocellular lipid (IMCL) content, visceral fat content, and hepatic fat content than their age, gender, and BMI matched pairs.[47] These obese young people with impaired glucose tolerance have a pronounced defect

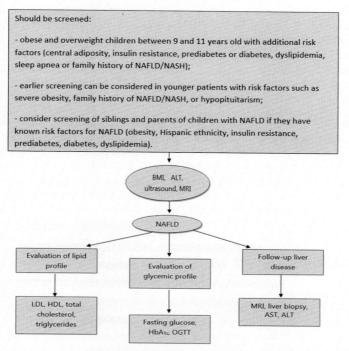

Should be screened:

- obese and overweight children between 9 and 11 years old with additional risk factors (central adiposity, insulin resistance, prediabetes or diabetes, dyslipidemia, sleep apnea or family history of NAFLD/NASH);

- earlier screening can be considered in younger patients with risk factors such as severe obesity, family history of NAFLD/NASH, or hypopituitarism;

- consider screening of siblings and parents of children with NAFLD if they have known risk factors for NAFLD (obesity, Hispanic ethnicity, insulin resistance, prediabetes, diabetes, dyslipidemia).

BMI, ALT, ultrasound, MRI

NAFLD

Evaluation of lipid profile → LDL, HDL, total cholesterol, triglycerides

Evaluation of glycemic profile → Fasting glucose, HbA1c, OGTT

Follow-up liver disease → MRI, liver biopsy, AST, ALT

FIG. 11.2 Recommendation for the screening of at risk obese children and adolescents.

in the nonoxidative pathway of glucose metabolism.[47] These events occur not only in the skeletal muscle, but also in the liver contributing to hepatic insulin resistance.[10] Hepatic insulin resistance is one of the primary disturbances responsible for the metabolic changes that occur in obese individuals and eventually leads to type 2 diabetes.[7,10]

β-CELL IMPAIRMENT IS THE LAST STEP BEFORE DEVELOPMENT OF TYPE 2 DIABETES

The relationship between insulin demand and secretion is a key factor regulating the maintenance of normal glucose tolerance. In fact, the β-cell responds to insulin resistance occurring in obese children and adolescents by producing a state of hyperinsulinemia, which maintains normal glucose levels.[48] In the long run, however, some individuals have deteriorating β-cell function, and insulin secretion may not be sufficient to maintain glucose levels within the normal range.[47–49]

In fact, when insulin secretion is estimated in the context of the "resistant milieu", IGT subjects show a significantly lower degree of insulin secretion than the group with a normal glucose tolerance (NGT).[47] In particular, using hyperglycemic clamp studies, Weiss et al.

investigated the role of insulin secretion in glucose regulation in a group of 62 obese adolescents with varying states of glucose tolerance (30 NGT, 22 IGT, and 10 type 2 diabetes).[50] This study showed that in comparison to NGT obese adolescents with similar insulin resistance, those with IGT show a progressive loss of glucose sensitivity of β-cell first-phase secretion and that the β-cell second-phase secretion is compromised in T2D.[50] This does not mean that the defect in the first phase is less influential than the defect of the second phase in causing hyperglycemia, yet simply recognizes that the decline of the first phase of the insulin secretion is present before overt diabetes and it may be considered the fingerprint of prediabetes, whereas the defect in the second phase is required for the development of type 2 diabetes. In fact, differences in β-cell function have been described in various prediabetic conditions seen in obese adolescents, such as impaired fasting glucose (IFG) or IGT, or the combined IFG/IGT states.[51,52] Cali et al. documented that in obese adolescents (1) IFG is primarily linked to alterations in glucose sensitivity of first-phase insulin secretion; (2) IGT is characterized by a more severe degree of peripheral insulin resistance and reduction in first-phase secretion; (3) the cooccurrence of IFG and IGT is the result of a defect in second-phase insulin secretion and a profound insulin resistance.[52]

In addition, genetic predisposition plays an important role in the development of type 2 diabetes. This idea is supported by clinical studies showing that youths developing IGT or T2D have less insulin secretion even before the onset of IGT or T2D.[52]

It is worth mentioning that changes in insulin secretion and sensitivity occur at a faster rate in youth than in adults. Although in adults the transition to type 2 diabetes takes about 10 years,[50] in obese youth it has been estimated that β-cell function reduction occurs at a rate of 15% per year,[50] with a mean transition time from prediabetes to overt diabetes of around 2.5 years. It means that type 2 diabetes in youth might be a more severe disease than in adults.

Please see Chapter 1 for More Information on the Pathophysiology of Insulin Resistance and T2D

TREATMENT OF NAFLD: WHERE ARE WE NOW?

The lack of long-term follow-up studies reporting the natural history of NAFLD in children makes highly controversial the selection of target population for treatment of NAFLD as well as for monitoring the actual efficacy of the therapeutic option.

There are no effective drugs, to date, for the treatment of NAFLD, however lifestyle interventions have been proved to be effective in slowing NASH progression and reverting NAFLD phenotype. They include dietary directions and physical activity and are mandatory in all the children with NAFLD. There is evidence for an effect on NAFLD regression from three main lifestyle interventions[40,53]:

- The consumption of a well-balanced diet for age[53];
- Avoidance of sweetener beverage[54];
- Regular physical exercise, for its effect on both BMI and fatty liver along with an improvement, over time, of insulin sensitivity[55];

There are no drugs currently labeled for treatment of NAFLD in pediatrics age, but several medications have been investigated attempting to revert or slowing down the progression from NALFD to NASH.

Antioxidants, by reducing oxidative stress, protect susceptible components of biological membranes from lipid peroxidation, and may, therefore, prevent the progression of simple steatosis to NASH. The most studied antioxidant in children with NAFLD is α-tocopherol (vitamin E) and warrants consideration in obesity-related liver dysfunction for children unable to adhere to low-calorie diets. In particular, Sanyal et al. showed that vitamin E therapy, as compared with placebo, was associated with a significantly higher rate of improvement in NASH (43% vs. 19%, $P = .001$) in adults without diabetes. For its pathogenic role, insulin resistance appears as an adequate therapeutic target. Metformin is the only insulin-sensitizing agent evaluated in children.

Lavine et al., in a more recent large, multicenter, randomized double-bind placebo-controlled trial (TONIC study), evaluated the effect of daily dosing of 800 IU of vitamin E (58 patients), 1000 mg of metformin (57 patients), or placebo (58 patients) for 96 weeks of NAFLD course. The patients (aged 8–17 years) with biopsy-confirmed NAFLD and persistently elevated levels of ALT, without diabetes or cirrhosis, were randomly assigned to 1 of 3 groups. At 96 weeks, neither vitamin E nor metformin was superior to placebo in attaining the primary outcome of sustained reduction in ALT level in pediatric NAFLD; vitamin E and metformin groups, however, showed an improvement in histological hepatocellular ballooning in NAFLD an NASH.[56]

Another, single-arm, open-label, small pilot study on metformin (500 mg twice daily for 24 weeks), conducted in 10 nondiabetic children with biopsy proven NASH and elevated ALT levels showed reduction of hepatic steatosis, as evaluated with magnetic resonance spectroscopy (MRS) and serum ALT concentrations.[57]

As mentioned previously, one of the effects of dysbiosis associated with NAFLD is the reduction in GLP-1 secretion from the intestinal L-cells. GLP-1 is a pleiotropic peptide, acting both centrally by inhibiting the appetite and on the β- and α-cells, as secretagogue for insulin and inhibitor for glucagon response. Indeed, GLP-1 analogues represent a promising therapeutic option for subjects with type 2 diabetes and, more recently, they seem to be effective in blunting the postprandial glucose peak also in type 1 diabetes by delaying gastric emptying.[58-61] GLP-1 might be beneficial for NAFLD, as well.[62] In fact, liraglutide, an analogue of GLP-1, has been demonstrated to lead to histological resolution of NASH in adults. The observed result, however, might be, at least partially, attributed to the effect of liraglutide on weight and glucose tolerance that could secondary determinate a benefit on fat liver accumulation.[62] It has to be indicated that not all the data in the literature support a beneficial effect of GLP-1 analogues in ameliorating NAFLD/NASH phenotype.[63]

CONCLUSIONS

NAFLD is a major public health problem among obese children and a major determinant of hepatic insulin resistance. The efforts in understanding its pathogenesis might help clinicians in preventing and treating this disease. However, although some studies have clearly helped understanding some of the mechanisms underlying its pathogenesis, these findings are far from being translated in clinical practice. Moreover, current clinical trials have failed to indicate a clear pharmacotherapy for NAFLD/NASH and its complications. Therefore more effort is essential to better evaluate the predisposition to NAFLD, the mechanisms through which gene variants, food quality, and other environmental factors lead to NAFLD and how we could leverage this knowledge to provide a cure to kids with NAFLD.

REFERENCES

1. Doulberis M, Kotronis G, Gialamprinou D, Kountouras J, Katsinelos P. Non-alcoholic fatty liver disease: an update with special focus on the role of gut microbiota. *Metabolism.* 2017;71:182–197.
2. Selvakumar PKC, Kabbany MN, Nobili V, Alkhouri N. Nonalcoholic fatty liver disease in children: hepatic and extrahepatic complications. *Pediatr Clin North Am.* 2017;64(3):659–675.
3. Guerrero R, Vega GL, Grundy SM, Browning JD. Ethnic differences in hepatic steatosis: an insulin resistance paradox? *Hepatology.* 2009;49(3):791–801.
4. Marzuillo P, Miraglia del Giudice E, Santoro N. Pediatric fatty liver disease: role of ethnicity and genetics. *World J Gastroenterol.* 2014;20(23):7347–7355.
5. Santoro N, Feldstein AE, Enoksson E, et al. The association between hepatic fat content and liver injury in obese children and adolescents: effects of ethnicity, insulin resistance, and common gene variants. *Diabetes Care.* 2013;36(5):1353–1360.
6. Browning JD, Szczepaniak LS, Dobbins R, et al. Prevalence of hepatic steatosis in an urban population in the United States: impact of ethnicity. *Hepatology.* 2004;40(6): 1387–1395.
7. Cali AM, De Oliveira AM, Kim H, et al. Glucose dysregulation and hepatic steatosis in obese adolescents: is there a link? *Hepatology.* 2009;49(6):1896–1903.
8. Newton KP, Hou J, Crimmins NA, et al. Prevalence of prediabetes and type 2 diabetes in children with nonalcoholic fatty liver disease. *JAMA Pediatr.* 2016;170(10):e161971.
9. Tilg H, Moschen AR, Roden M. NAFLD and diabetes mellitus. *Nat Rev Gastroenterol Hepatol.* 2017;14(1):32–42.
10. D'Adamo E, Cali AM, Weiss R, et al. Central role of fatty liver in the pathogenesis of insulin resistance in obese adolescents. *Diabetes Care.* 2010;33(8):1817–1822.
11. Erion DM, Shulman GI. Diacylglycerol-mediated insulin resistance. *Nat Med.* 2010;16(4):400–402.
12. Roden M. Mechanisms of Disease: hepatic steatosis in type 2 diabetes–pathogenesis and clinical relevance. *Nat Clin Pract Endocrinol Metab.* 2006;2(6):335–348.
13. Ouchi N, Parker JL, Lugus JJ, Walsh K. Adipokines in inflammation and metabolic disease. *Nat Rev Immunol.* 2011;11(2):85–97.
14. Taksali SE, Caprio S, Dziura J, et al. High visceral and low abdominal subcutaneous fat stores in the obese adolescent: a determinant of an adverse metabolic phenotype. *Diabetes.* 2008;57(2):367–371.
15. Haas JT, Francque S, Staels B. Pathophysiology and mechanisms of nonalcoholic fatty liver disease. *Annu Rev Physiol.* 2016;78:181–205.
16. Moschen AR, Kaser S, Tilg H. Non-alcoholic steatohepatitis: a microbiota-driven disease. *Trends Endocrinol Metab.* 2013;24(11):537–545.
17. Lambert JE, Ramos-Roman MA, Browning JD, Parks EJ. Increased de novo lipogenesis is a distinct characteristic of individuals with nonalcoholic fatty liver disease. *Gastroenterology.* 2014;146(3):726–735.
18. Donnelly KL, Smith CI, Schwarzenberg SJ, Jessurun J, Boldt MD, Parks EJ. Sources of fatty acids stored in liver and secreted via lipoproteins in patients with nonalcoholic fatty liver disease. *J Clin Investig.* 2005;115(5):1343–1351.
19. Dentin R, Girard J, Postic C. Carbohydrate responsive element binding protein (ChREBP) and sterol regulatory element binding protein-1c (SREBP-1c): two key regulators of glucose metabolism and lipid synthesis in liver. *Biochimie.* 2005;87(1):81–86.
20. Speliotes EK, Yerges-Armstrong LM, Wu J, et al. Genome-wide association analysis identifies variants associated with nonalcoholic fatty liver disease that have distinct effects on metabolic traits. *PLoS Genet.* 2011;7(3):e1001324.
21. Santoro N, Kursawe R, D'Adamo E, et al. A common variant in the patatin-like phospholipase 3 gene (PNPLA3) is associated with fatty liver disease in obese children and adolescents. *Hepatology.* 2010;52(4):1281–1290.
22. Kozlitina J, Smagris E, Stender S, et al. Exome-wide association study identifies a TM6SF2 variant that confers susceptibility to nonalcoholic fatty liver disease. *Nat Genet.* 2014;46(4):352–356.
23. Huang Y, Cohen JC, Hobbs HH. Expression and characterization of a PNPLA3 protein isoform (I148M) associated with nonalcoholic fatty liver disease. *J Biol Chem.* 2011;286(43):37085–37093.
24. Saxena R, Voight BF, Lyssenko V, et al. Genome-wide association analysis identifies loci for type 2 diabetes and triglyceride levels. *Science.* 2007;316(5829):1331–1336.
25. Willer CJ, Sanna S, Jackson AU, et al. Newly identified loci that influence lipid concentrations and risk of coronary artery disease. *Nat Genet.* 2008;40(2):161–169.
26. Beer NL, Tribble ND, McCulloch LJ, et al. The P446L variant in GCKR associated with fasting plasma glucose and triglyceride levels exerts its effect through increased glucokinase activity in liver. *Hum Mol Genet.* 2009;18(21):4081–4088.
27. Goffredo M, Caprio S, Feldstein AE, et al. Role of TM6SF2 rs58542926 in the pathogenesis of nonalcoholic pediatric fatty liver disease: a multiethnic study. *Hepatology.* 2016;63(1):117–125.

28. Umano GR, Martino M, Santoro N. The association between pediatric NAFLD and common genetic variants. *Child (Basel)*. 2017;4(6).

29. Mis NF, Braegger C, Bronsky J, et al. Sugar in infants, children and adolescents: a position paper of the European Society for Paediatric Gastroenterology, Hepatology and Nutrition Committee on Nutrition. *J Pediatr Gastroenterol Nutr*. 2017.

30. Kursawe R, Eszlinger M, Narayan D, et al. Cellularity and adipogenic profile of the abdominal subcutaneous adipose tissue from obese adolescents: association with insulin resistance and hepatic steatosis. *Diabetes*. 2010;59(9):2288–2296.

31. Schwarz JM, Noworolski SM, Erkin-Cakmak A, et al. Effects of dietary fructose restriction on liver fat, de novo lipogenesis, and insulin kinetics in children with obesity. *Gastroenterology*. 2017;153(3):743–752.

32. Wei X, Song M, Yin X, et al. Effects of dietary different doses of copper and high fructose feeding on rat fecal metabolome. *J Proteome Res*. 2015;14(9):4050–4058.

33. Wagnerberger S, Spruss A, Kanuri G, et al. Toll-like receptors 1-9 are elevated in livers with fructose-induced hepatic steatosis. *Br J Nutr*. 2012;107(12):1727–1738.

34. Lambertz J, Weiskirchen S, Landert S, Weiskirchen R. Fructose: a dietary sugar in crosstalk with microbiota contributing to the development and progression of non-alcoholic liver disease. *Front Immunol*. 2017;8:1159.

35. Wigg AJ, Roberts-Thomson IC, Dymock RB, McCarthy PJ, Grose RH, Cummins AG. The role of small intestinal bacterial overgrowth, intestinal permeability, endotoxaemia, and tumour necrosis factor alpha in the pathogenesis of non-alcoholic steatohepatitis. *Gut*. 2001;48(2):206–211.

36. Leung C, Rivera L, Furness JB, Angus PW. The role of the gut microbiota in NAFLD. *Nat Rev Gastroenterol Hepatol*. 2016;13(7):412–425.

37. Goffredo M, Mass K, Parks EJ, et al. Role of gut microbiota and short chain fatty acids in modulating energy harvest and fat partitioning in youth. *J Clin Endocrinol Metab*. 2016;101(11):4367–4376.

38. Wong RJ, Cheung R, Ahmed A. Nonalcoholic steatohepatitis is the most rapidly growing indication for liver transplantation in patients with hepatocellular carcinoma in the US. *Hepatology*. 2014;59(6):2188–2195.

39. Spencer MD, Hamp TJ, Reid RW, Fischer LM, Zeisel SH, Fodor AA. Association between composition of the human gastrointestinal microbiome and development of fatty liver with choline deficiency. *Gastroenterology*. 2011;140(3):976–986.

40. Vos MB, Abrams SH, Barlow SE, et al. NASPGHAN clinical practice guideline for the diagnosis and treatment of nonalcoholic fatty liver disease in children: recommendations from the expert committee on NAFLD (ECON) and the North American Society of Pediatric Gastroenterology, Hepatology and Nutrition (NASPGHAN). *J Pediatr Gastroenterol Nutr*. 2017;64(2):319–334.

41. Schwimmer JB, Newton KP, Awai HI, et al. Paediatric gastroenterology evaluation of overweight and obese children referred from primary care for suspected nonalcoholic fatty liver disease. *Aliment Pharmacol Ther*. 2013;38(10):1267–1277.

42. Nobili V, Vizzutti F, Arena U, et al. Accuracy and reproducibility of transient elastography for the diagnosis of fibrosis in pediatric nonalcoholic steatohepatitis. *Hepatology*. 2008;48(2):442–448.

43. Xanthakos SA, Podberesky DJ, Serai SD, et al. Use of magnetic resonance elastography to assess hepatic fibrosis in children with chronic liver disease. *J Pediatr*. 2014;164(1):186–188.

44. Venkatesh SK, Yin M, Ehman RL. Magnetic resonance elastography of liver: technique, analysis, and clinical applications. *J Magn Reson Imag*. 2013;37(3):544–555.

45. Venkatesh SK, Wells ML, Miller FH, et al. Magnetic resonance elastography: beyond liver fibrosis-a case-based pictorial review. *Abdom Radiol*. 2017.

46. Brunt EM, Kleiner DE, Wilson LA, Belt P, Neuschwander-Tetri BA. (CRN) NCRN. Nonalcoholic fatty liver disease (NAFLD) activity score and the histopathologic diagnosis in NAFLD: distinct clinicopathologic meanings. *Hepatology*. 2011;53(3):810–820.

47. Weiss R, Dufour S, Taksali SE, et al. Prediabetes in obese youth: a syndrome of impaired glucose tolerance, severe insulin resistance, and altered myocellular and abdominal fat partitioning. *Lancet*. 2003;362(9388):951–957.

48. Weiss R, Caprio S, Trombetta M, Taksali SE, Tamborlane WV, Bonadonna R. Beta-cell function across the spectrum of glucose tolerance in obese youth. *Diabetes*. 2005;54(6):1735–1743.

49. Weiss R, Cali AM, Dziura J, Burgert TS, Tamborlane WV, Caprio S. Degree of obesity and glucose allostasis are major effectors of glucose tolerance dynamics in obese youth. *Diabetes Care*. 2007;30(7):1845–1850.

50. Weiss R, Taksali SE, Tamborlane WV, Burgert TS, Savoye M, Caprio S. Predictors of changes in glucose tolerance status in obese youth. *Diabetes Care*. 2005;28(4):902–909.

51. Cali AM, Bonadonna RC, Trombetta M, Weiss R, Caprio S. Metabolic abnormalities underlying the different prediabetic phenotypes in obese adolescents. *J Clin Endocrinol Metabol*. 2008;93(5):1767–1773.

52. Cali AM, Man CD, Cobelli C, et al. Primary defects in beta-cell function further exacerbated by worsening of insulin resistance mark the development of impaired glucose tolerance in obese adolescents. *Diabetes Care*. 2009;32(3):456–461.

53. Nadeau KJ, Ehlers LB, Zeitler PS, Love-Osborne K. Treatment of non-alcoholic fatty liver disease with metformin versus lifestyle intervention in insulin-resistant adolescents. *Pediatr Diabetes*. 2009;10(1):5–13.

54. de Ruyter JC, Olthof MR, Seidell JC, Katan MB. A trial of sugar-free or sugar-sweetened beverages and body weight in children. *N Engl J Med*. 2012;367(15):1397–1406.

55. Lee S, Bacha F, Hannon T, Kuk JL, Boesch C, Arslanian S. Effects of aerobic versus resistance exercise without caloric restriction on abdominal fat, intrahepatic lipid, and insulin sensitivity in obese adolescent boys: a randomized, controlled trial. *Diabetes*. 2012;61(11): 2787–2795.

56. Lavine JE, Schwimmer JB, Van Natta ML, et al. Effect of vitamin E or metformin for treatment of nonalcoholic fatty liver disease in children and adolescents: the TONIC randomized controlled trial. *JAMA The Journal Am Med Assoc*. 2011;305(16):1659–1668.

57. Nobili V, Manco M, Ciampalini P, et al. Metformin use in children with nonalcoholic fatty liver disease: an open-label, 24-month, observational pilot study. *Clin Therapeut*. 2008;30(6):1168–1176.

58. Kramer CK, Zinman B, Choi H, Connelly PW, Retnakaran R. The impact of chronic liraglutide therapy on glucagon secretion in type 2 diabetes: insight from the LIBRA trial. *J Clin Endocrinol Metab*. 2015;100(10): 3702–3709.

59. Kaku K, Kiyosue A, Ono Y, et al. Liraglutide is effective and well tolerated in combination with an oral antidiabetic drug in Japanese patients with type 2 diabetes: a randomized, 52-week, open-label, parallel-group trial. *J Diabetes Investig*. 2016;7(1):76–84.

60. Bode BW, Garg SK. The Emerging role of Adjunctive Non-insulin Antihyperglycemic therapy in the Management of type 1 diabetes. *Endocr Pract*. 2016;22(2):220–230.

61. Dejgaard TF, Frandsen CS, Hansen TS, et al. Efficacy and safety of liraglutide for overweight adult patients with type 1 diabetes and insufficient glycaemic control (Lira-1): a randomised, double-blind, placebo-controlled trial. *Lancet Diabetes Endocrinol*. 2016;4(3):221–232.

62. Petit JM, Cercueil JP, Loffroy R, et al. Effect of liraglutide therapy on liver fat content in patients with inadequately controlled type 2 diabetes: the Lira-NAFLD study. *J Clin Endocrinol Metabol*. 2017;102(2):407–415.

63. Smits MM, Tonneijck L, Muskiet MH, et al. Twelve week liraglutide or sitagliptin does not affect hepatic fat in type 2 diabetes: a randomised placebo-controlled trial. *Diabetologia*. 2016;59(12):2588–2593.

CHAPTER 12

Medications for the Treatment of Type II Diabetes

MICHELLE A. VAN NAME, MD

INTRODUCTION

Other than the TODAY study,[1] there have been few studies that evaluate medical therapy in adolescents with type 2 diabetes (T2D), thus expert opinion frames much of pediatric diabetes management. For initial treatment of youth who may have T2D, the severity of hyperglycemia and metabolic decompensation at the time of diagnosis dictates the treatment. For pediatric patients who are asymptomatic, often diagnosed on routine screening, and who have only modest elevations in HbA1c and plasma glucose, metformin is the standard initial therapy. For patients in whom type 1 diabetes is being considered, insulin should be initiated. This is especially prudent in those with serum blood glucose $\geq$250 mg/dL or HbA1c >9%.[2] Once a child on insulin is clinically diagnosed with T2D, metformin should be added and insulin may be weaned if this is reasonable based on glycemic control. Newly diagnosed youth often have considerable improvement in glycemic control once started on insulin and metformin. This allows for the insulin doses to be weaned off and stopped, after which the patient is maintained on metformin monotherapy.

METFORMIN

Metformin is in the biguanide class of medications and has been available for more than 60 years. Despite its extensive history in treatment of T2D and use in both children and adults, research continues to elucidate the mechanisms by which metformin may impact glucose metabolism. In addition to decreasing hepatic glucose production, metformin improves hepatic insulin sensitivity, affects the gut microbiome, increases glucagon-like peptide (GLP-1), and decreases inflammation.[3]

Currently, metformin remains the only noninsulin medication approved for treatment of T2D in youth. Metformin is the standard treatment, and the treatment to which other diabetes medications are added unless the patient has a contraindication to metformin use.

Therapy with metformin is superior to placebo in youth with T2D[4]; however, the TODAY study found that metformin alone does not adequately sustain glycemic control in most youth.[1] On further analysis, it was identified that those adolescents who were unable to maintain an HbA1c below the diabetes range were more likely to have a rapid progression of diabetes with loss of glycemic control on metformin alone.[5] Thus, metformin monotherapy may be a more durable treatment for those adolescents with lower HbA1c at baseline.

Administration

Prior to administration, renal function should be assessed as metformin is cleared by the kidneys, and should not be used if GFR $\leq$45 mL/min/1.73 m^2. Renal function should be monitored annually. Prior to prescribing, it is also reasonable to assess for hepatic impairment, as this can contribute to impaired clearance of lactate.[6]

To begin metformin therapy, the metformin is slowly titrated up to a goal maximal dose of 2000 mg per day.[2] Immediate release metformin is available in 500, 850, and 1000 mg tablets and in a 500 mg/5 mL oral solution. To mitigate gastrointestinal side effects, metformin is typically initiated at a dose of 500 mg with breakfast or dinner daily. A second dose is added at the other meal after 1 week, or longer if gastrointestinal side effects have not resolved at 1 week. Additional doses are added weekly, or after lengthier duration if needed, until patients are taking 1000 mg with breakfast and 1000 mg with dinner. Not all patients are able to titrate up to this dose.

An extended release formulation is also available, in tablets of 500, 750, and 1000 mg. The extended release formulation has fewer gastrointestinal side effects than the immediate release formulation,[7] and is dosed the same way. The extended release tablets provide an

Pediatric Type II Diabetes. https://doi.org/10.1016/B978-0-323-55138-0.00012-7

alternate treatment strategy for patients who cannot tolerate the side effects of immediate release metformin, do not routinely eat breakfast, or who have difficulty taking medication twice a day. For adolescents who rush to get to school in the morning, it may not be realistic to reliably take oral medication and eat. In these cases, clinicians often titrate up to a once daily dose of 1500 mg (can be taken as two 750 mg tabs) or 2000 mg extended release metformin.

Given the strong family history of T2D in many of the youth with this diagnosis, parents and teens can be encouraged to take their prescribed metformin together, to ensure supervision of medication administration.

Side Effects/Considerations

Patients should be counseled regarding the expected side effects of metformin treatment, including abdominal discomfort, nausea, and diarrhea. These effects can be mitigated by dosing metformin with meals, and with continued stable dosing these side effects should cease.

Lactic acidosis has been described in the setting of renal impairment and decline in renal function due to receiving IV contrast, age ≥65 years, congestive heart failure, excessive alcohol intake, and hepatic impairment.[6] Metformin should be held during periods of poor or no oral intake. Long-term use of metformin has been associated with vitamin B12 deficiency in adults,[8] thus clinicians may consider routine monitoring of vitamin B12 and/or prophylactic treatment with a multivitamin. Some weight loss effects have been reported with use of metformin in adolescents with overweight/obesity.[9,10]

INSULIN

As noted earlier, insulin is indicated when the distinction between type 1 and type 2 diabetes is unclear, or when significant hyperglycemia is present in the setting of metformin monotherapy. A typical starting dose for insulin ranges from 0.75 to 1.25 units/kg/day, but with titration doses may reach 2 units/kg/day or more. Currently, research is ongoing to determine whether prompt insulin initiation restores β-cell function in early T2D in youth.[11]

Basal Insulins

In contrast to youth with T1D, youth with T2D may require basal insulin only to achieve targeted glycemic control. Initial dosing of 0.25–0.5 units/kg of basal insulin can be started and titrated as necessary.[12] Commonly used basal insulins and their duration

of action at standard concentrations include insulin detemir (14–21 h), insulin glargine (>24 h), and insulin degludec (>42 h).[13] Basal insulin may be started at diagnosis (see introduction) or added onto metformin therapy if glycemic targets are not met.

Concentrated insulins are a helpful tool to address the high doses of insulin that may be required in youth with T2D. Insulin glargine pens are available in a 300 unit/mL concentration, and insulin degludec pens are available in a 200 unit/mL concentration. Although glargine 300 unit/mL has a longer duration of action and more consistent profile compared to glargine 100 units/mL,[14] degludec U100 and U200 have similar properties.[15]

The higher insulin dosage that can be administered in a single injection of concentrated formulations may be more realistic to optimize compliance in adolescents than administration of multiple basal insulin doses, although there is a paucity of evidence on their usage in children and adolescents. Safety measures are essential when using nonstandard insulin concentrations. There is concern for more clinically significant episodes of hypoglycemia.

Bolus Insulins

If HbA1c goals (<6.5%) are not reached with basal insulin alone, clinicians should add bolus insulin to the regimen.[12] Bolus insulins include insulins aspart, lispro, and glulisine. Insulin lispro is available in a concentrated 200 unit/mL form. Dosing of short acting insulin should be individualized to the patient's needs. Specific bolus dosage recommendations are lacking in this population. Clinicians can consider utilizing weight (initial bolus dose of 0.1 units/kg),[16] basal dose (10% of basal dose),[16] or flat dosing (we often begin with 10–20 units at mealtime) when initiating bolus dosing. Frequent phone contact with rapid titration to therapeutic dosages may be necessary. Youth may require bolus dosing only for the largest meal of the day, although when bolus dosing is essential we find that adolescents often require it for all meals consumed. Importantly, in youth with T2D who maintain some β-cell function, finely titrated bolus dosing may not be required because endogenous insulin production can help manage postprandial hyperglycemia. Simplified dosing, for example 30 units of short acting or bolus insulin with each meal, may be preferable and a more realistic management plan for some adolescents.

Furthermore, mixed insulins are often used in adolescents with T2D. These mixed insulins allow for dosing of short/intermediate acting insulin 1–2 times per day. Residual β-cell function can compensate for insulin to glucose mismatch that occurs in the absence of dedicated bolus insulin. Mixed insulins are especially valuable in managing diabetes in youth in whom adherence to a basal bolus schedule is a challenge and in those youth who eat intermittently throughout the day. Additionally, one can consider use of a newer insulin degludec/insulin aspart mix.

Weaning

Insulin can be weaned based on glycemic control as well as HbA1c targets. Bolus insulin is usually weaned off first, followed by basal insulin. Particular attention should be given to weaning of insulin during up-titration of metformin dosing, and based on success of lifestyle intervention and changes in body composition.

OTHER AGENTS BEING INVESTIGATED IN PEDIATRIC STUDIES

Newer pharmacologic agents, including sodium-glucose cotransporter (SGLT) 2 inhibitors and GLP-1 receptor agonists, which are approved for use in adults with T2D, are currently being studied in youth with T2D. Although these are not FDA approved for use in pediatric patients at this time, we anticipate that approvals for some of these newer agents will be forthcoming and applicable to management strategies in the future. Furthermore, the weight loss side effects of some agents is an appealing attribute for use in pediatric T2D. Additional medications such as dipeptidyl peptidase 4 (DPP-4) inhibitors are weight neutral and being studied in adolescents. When adding on an additional agent to the regimen for patients who are on insulin, blood glucose should be monitored regularly so that insulin dosing can be decreased if warranted.

GLP-1 Receptor Agonists

GLP-1 agonists have become available in recent years. These agents activate GLP-1 receptors, which lead to improved glucose-mediated insulin secretion while decreasing glucagon secretion, slow gastric emptying, and promote satiety. Injectable GLP-1 agonists include BID exenatide, daily liraglutide and lixisenatide, and weekly albiglutide, dulaglutide, and exenatide. Semaglutide is under evaluation by the FDA and has an oral formulation as well. Combination agents available include insulin degludec + liraglutide, as well as insulin glargine + lixisenatide.

In adults with T2D, GLP-1 agonist therapy decreases HbA1c by about 1%[17] and weight by about 2.8 kg.[18] A randomized trial of 846 adults with T2D[19] resulted in weight loss of ≥5% in 54.3% of participants taking liraglutide 3.0 mg and 40.4% of those on liraglutide

1.8 mg, with overall weight loss of 6.5 kg (6%) at the 3.0 mg dose and 5 kg (4.7%) at the 1.8 mg dose. HbA1c decreased by 1.3% and 1.1% with these dosages, respectively. Pediatric studies are ongoing for multiple GLP-1 agonists. A prior study evaluated exenatide in youth with severe obesity, and has provided preliminary evidence of safety in a pediatric population.[20]

As one may anticipate based on the mechanism of action of this incretin mimetic, side effects of GLP-1 agonist therapy include nausea, vomiting, and diarrhea, and they have a low risk of hypoglycemia. Satiety effects contribute to weight loss. Recent trials have not found an increased risk of pancreatitis in the setting of GLP-1 agonist use.[21-24] Rodent studies have reported that GLP-1 receptor activation promotes C cell hyperplasia and medullary thyroid cancer[24]; however, this conclusion has not been reached in human studies. Personal or family history of medullary thyroid cancer should be solicited prior to prescribing a GLP-1 receptor agonist.

An additional consideration is the impact of GLP-1 receptor agonists on comorbidities associated with T2D. Drugs from this class have been shown to prevent diabetic nephropathy[25] and improve cardiovascular outcomes[21,22] in adults with T2D.

DPP-4 Inhibitors

Dipeptidyl peptidase-4 is an enzyme that deactivates GLP-1 and other peptides. Thus, inhibition of DPP-4 should increase availability of intrinsic GLP-1 and result in the effects described earlier, although they are not associated with weight loss. DPP-4 inhibitors are oral agents that have been available since 2006 to treat adults with T2D.[26] Current agents include alogliptin, linagliptin, saxagliptin, sitagliptin, and vildagliptin (this agent is not available in the United States).

To date, there have been limited studies of DPP-4 inhibitors completed in pediatric patients with T2D. Pharmacokinetics and dynamics were found to be similar in children and adolescents with T2D when compared to adults.[27] A small phase IIb study found the safety and efficacy of linagliptin to be similar in pediatric patients to that described in adults.[28] The decrement in HbA1c at 12 weeks was 0.48% for the 1 mg dose and 0.63% for the 5 mg dose. Additional studies are ongoing or planned.

DPP-4 inhibitors tend to be well tolerated with minimal side effects, including little impact on weight. Concerns have arisen regarding pancreatitis; however, assessment of the data has concluded no causality of DPP-4 inhibitors to trigger pancreatitis.[29]

Multiple DPP-4 inhibitors have completed large evaluations of cardiovascular safety and were found to have no impact on ischemic cardiovascular events.[30-33]

Although the study of saxagliptin found a small increase in hospitalizations for heart failure,[30] this was not confirmed in other studies.[31-33]

SGLT Inhibitors

Sodium–glucose cotransporter 2 inhibitors act by limiting glucose reabsorption in the kidney at a lower threshold through inhibition of SGLT2 in the distal nephron. This causes renal glucosuria, resulting in lower blood glucose. Currently available agents include canagliflozin, dapagliflozin, and empagliflozin. Sotagliflozin is a combined SGLT1 and 2 inhibitor that is not yet available.

SGLT2 inhibitors have been studied extensively in adults with T2D, and have been shown to decrease HbA1c by 0.9%-0.6%.[34] Pediatric studies are underway to determine whether this treatment option is appropriate for youth with T2D.

SGLT2 inhibitors have side effects of weight loss and lower blood pressure. Adverse side effects include polyuria and potential for volume depletion, as well as genitourinary infections. There is also potential for ketosis in the setting of lowered insulin dose due to more effective glucose regulation while on SGLT2 inhibitor therapy. This relative insulinopenia in the presence of a stress allows for increased lipolysis, which releases substrates for ketone production.[35] This can progress to diabetic ketoacidosis, which has been reported in patients with T1D and also in patients with T2D.

In a large randomized controlled trial, empagliflozin has decreased major adverse cardiovascular events,[36] a benefit that was unprecedented with use of diabetes medications.[37] Although studies examining the effect of dapagliflozin and canagliflozin on renal outcomes are underway, treatment of adults with T2D with empagliflozin has already been shown to reduce the risk of nephropathy.[38]

Rapid Acting Bromocriptine

Bromocriptine is a dopamine-2 agonist and FDA indicated for treatment of type 2 diabetes in adults. Morning administration of this oral medication activates the D2 receptor, which maintains hypothalamic neural activities to mitigate peripheral insulin resistance, hepatic glucose production, as well as lipolysis of adipose tissue.[39] Nondiabetic individuals have increased dopaminergic activity in the morning[39]; thus, this medication improves fasting as well as postprandial blood glucose values.[40] Treatment with rapid acting bromocriptine reduces HbA1c by about 0.6%.[41] A pharmacokinetic study has been completed in youth with T2D.

Side effects include gastrointestinal symptoms of nausea, vomiting, and diarrhea and headache or dizziness have also been reported.[42] Bromocriptine is a weight neutral medication with a low risk of hypoglycemia.[40] There is evidence that use of bromocriptine in adults with T2D decreases cardiovascular events.[42]

OTHER AGENTS COMMONLY USED IN ADULT T2D

The agents below are also not approved for pediatric use, and have side effects that limit their desirability for use in pediatric patients. Patients with higher HbA1c have greater potential for magnitude of improvement with therapy intensification utilizing additional agents. HbA1c reduction tends to be more robust with metformin, GLP-1 receptor agonists, thiazolidinediones (TZDs), and sulfonylureas,[43] although the latter 2 are not currently being studied in youth.

Thiazolidinediones

TZDs work by activating peroxisome proliferator-activated receptor (PPARs), which are nuclear transcription factors. TZDs improve insulin sensitivity, and when used as monotherapy they are as effective as metformin in lowering HbA1c.[44] Currently available agents are pioglitazone and rosiglitazone.

The TODAY study of youth with T2D included a cohort that received metformin + rosiglitazone, and this group had longer durability of glycemic control than the groups received metformin alone or metformin with lifestyle modification.[1] In adults with T2D, TZDs lower HbA1c by about 1%-1.6%.[45,46]

Side effects of TZDs include weight gain, bone fractures, and increase in LDL,[47] as well as increased rates of heart failure.[48]

Sulfonylureas

Sulfonylureas (SU) work by acting at the β cell to close K_{ATP} channels, which increases insulin secretion. Currently available agents include glipizide, glyburide, and glimepiride. When used as monotherapy there is no difference compared to metformin.[49] Monotherapy with SU lowers HbA1c by about 1.5%.[50]

A major side effect of SU limiting their use is hypoglycemia. They are also associated with weight gain and may impair ischemic preconditioning.[43] Management with SUs lowers the risk of microvascular disease.[51]

CONCLUSION

Management of T2D in youth is very challenging. The current management tools available are limited, and there are often concerns regarding compliance in the setting of metformin side effects and insulin regimens.

As we continue to learn more about the pathophysiology of T2D in youth, studies are ongoing to increase the arsenal of medications that can be added to management with lifestyle modification. Newer insulins allow for more flexibility in design of treatment plans.

REFERENCES

1. Today Studdy Group, Zeitler P, Hirst K, et al. A clinical trial to maintain glycemic control in youth with type 2 diabetes. *N Engl J Med.* 2012;366(24):2247–2256.
2. Copeland KC, Silverstein J, Moore KR, et al. Management of newly diagnosed type 2 Diabetes Mellitus (T2DM) in children and adolescents. *Pediatrics.* 2013;131(2):364–382.
3. Rena G, Hardie DG, Pearson ER. The mechanisms of action of metformin. *Diabetologia.* 2017.
4. Jones KL, Arslanian S, Peterokova VA, Park JS, Tomlinson MJ. Effect of metformin in pediatric patients with type 2 diabetes: a randomized controlled trial. *Diabetes Care.* 2002;25(1):89–94.
5. Zeitler P, Hirst K, Copeland KC, et al. HbA1c after a short period of monotherapy with metformin Identifies durable glycemic control among adolescents with type 2 diabetes. *Diabetes Care.* 2015;38(12):2285–2292.
6. *Package Insert Glucophage® (Metformin Hydrochloride) Tablets Glucophage® XR (Metformin Hydrochloride) Extended-release Tablets.* 2017. https://packageinserts.bms.com/pi/pi_glucophage.pdf.
7. Fujita Y, Inagaki N. Metformin: new preparations and nonglycemic benefits. *Curr Diab Rep.* 2017;17(1):5.
8. Aroda VR, Edelstein SL, Goldberg RB, et al. Long-term metformin use and vitamin B12 deficiency in the diabetes prevention program outcomes study. *J Clin Endocrinol Metab.* 2016;101(4):1754–1761.
9. Kendall D, Vail A, Amin R, et al. Metformin in obese children and adolescents: the MOCA trial. *J Clin Endocrinol Metab.* 2013;98(1):322–329.
10. McDonagh MS, Selph S, Ozpinar A, Foley C. Systematic review of the benefits and risks of metformin in treating obesity in children aged 18 years and younger. *JAMA Pediatr.* 2014;168(2):178–184.
11. Consortium R. Restoring Insulin Secretion (RISE): design of studies of beta-cell preservation in prediabetes and early type 2 diabetes across the life span. *Diabetes Care.* 2014;37(3):780–788.
12. Zeitler P, Fu J, Tandon N, et al. ISPAD clinical practice consensus guidelines 2014. Type 2 diabetes in the child and adolescent. *Pediatr Diab.* 2014;15(suppl 20):26–46.
13. Lajara R, Cengiz E, Tanenberg RJ. The role of the new basal insulin analogs in addressing unmet clinical needs in people with type 1 and type 2 diabetes. *Curr Med Res Opin.* 2017;33(6):1045–1055.
14. Becker RH, Dahmen R, Bergmann K, Lehmann A, Jax T, Heise T. New insulin glargine 300 Units. mL-1 provides a more even activity profile and prolonged glycemic control at steady state compared with insulin glargine 100 Units mL-1. *Diabetes Care.* 2015;38(4):637–643.
15. Haahr H, Heise T. A review of the pharmacological properties of insulin degludec and their clinical relevance. *Clin Pharmacokinet.* 2014;53(9):787–800.
16. American Diabetes A. 8. Pharmacologic approaches to glycemic treatment: standards of medical care in Diabetes-2018. *Diabetes Care.* 2018;41(suppl 1):S73–S85.
17. Shyangdan DS, Royle P, Clar C, Sharma P, Waugh N, Snaith A. Glucagon-like peptide analogues for type 2 diabetes mellitus. *Cochrane Database Syst Rev.* 2011;(10):CD006423.
18. Vilsboll T, Christensen M, Junker AE, Knop FK, Gluud LL. Effects of glucagon-like peptide-1 receptor agonists on weight loss: systematic review and meta-analyses of randomised controlled trials. *BMJ.* 2012;344:d7771.
19. Davies MJ, Bergenstal R, Bode B, et al. Efficacy of liraglutide for weight loss among patients with type 2 diabetes: the SCALE diabetes randomized clinical trial. *JAMA.* 2015;314(7):687–699.
20. Kelly AS, Rudser KD, Nathan BM, et al. The effect of glucagon-like peptide-1 receptor agonist therapy on body mass index in adolescents with severe obesity: a randomized, placebo-controlled, clinical trial. *JAMA Pediatr.* 2013;167(4):355–360.
21. Marso SP, Bain SC, Consoli A, et al. Semaglutide and cardiovascular outcomes in patients with type 2 diabetes. *N Engl J Med.* 2016;375(19):1834–1844.
22. Marso SP, Daniels GH, Brown-Frandsen K, et al. Liraglutide and cardiovascular outcomes in type 2 diabetes. *N Engl J Med.* 2016;375(4):311–322.
23. Pfeffer MA, Claggett B, Diaz R, et al. Lixisenatide in patients with type 2 diabetes and acute coronary syndrome. *N Engl J Med.* 2015;373(23):2247–2257.
24. Drucker DJ, Sherman SI, Bergenstal RM, Buse JB. The safety of incretin-based therapies–review of the scientific evidence. *J Clin Endocrinol Metab.* 2011;96(7):2027–2031.
25. Mann JFE, Orsted DD, Brown-Frandsen K, et al. Liraglutide and renal outcomes in type 2 diabetes. *N Engl J Med.* 2017;377(9):839–848.
26. Deacon CF, Lebovitz HE. Comparative review of dipeptidyl peptidase-4 inhibitors and sulphonylureas. *Diab Obes Metab.* 2016;18(4):333–347.
27. Dudkowski C, Tsai M, Liu J, Zhao Z, Schmidt E, Xie J. The pharmacokinetics and pharmacodynamics of alogliptin in children, adolescents, and adults with type 2 diabetes mellitus. *Eur J Clin Pharmacol.* 2017;73(3):279–288.
28. Tamborlane WV, Laffel LM, Weill J, et al. Randomized, double-blind, placebo-controlled dose-finding study of the dipeptidyl peptidase-4 inhibitor linagliptin in pediatric patients with type 2 diabetes. *Pediatr Diab.* 2017.
29. Egan AG, Blind E, Dunder K, et al. Pancreatic safety of incretin-based drugs–FDA and EMA assessment. *N Engl J Med.* 2014;370(9):794–797.
30. Scirica BM, Bhatt DL, Braunwald E, et al. Saxagliptin and cardiovascular outcomes in patients with type 2 diabetes mellitus. *N Engl J Med.* 2013;369(14):1317–1326.

31. Zannad F, Cannon CP, Cushman WC, et al. Heart failure and mortality outcomes in patients with type 2 diabetes taking alogliptin versus placebo in EXAMINE: a multicentre, randomised, double-blind trial. *Lancet.* 2015;385(9982):2067–2076.

32. Gantz I, Chen M, Suryawanshi S, et al. A randomized, placebo-controlled study of the cardiovascular safety of the once-weekly DPP-4 inhibitor omarigliptin in patients with type 2 diabetes mellitus. *Cardiovasc Diabetol.* 2017;16(1):112.

33. Green JB, Bethel MA, Armstrong PW, et al. Effect of sitagliptin on cardiovascular outcomes in type 2 diabetes. *N Engl J Med.* 2015;373(3):232–242.

34. Zaccardi F, Webb DR, Htike ZZ, Youssef D, Khunti K, Davies MJ. Efficacy and safety of sodium-glucose co-transporter-2 inhibitors in type 2 diabetes mellitus: systematic review and network meta-analysis. *Diab Obes Metab.* 2016;18(8):783–794.

35. Monica Reddy RP, Inzucchi SE. SGLT2 inhibitors in the management of type 2 diabetes. *Endocrine.* 2016;53(2):364–372.

36. Zinman B, Wanner C, Lachin JM, et al. Empagliflozin, cardiovascular outcomes, and mortality in type 2 diabetes. *N Engl J Med.* 2015;373(22):2117–2128.

37. Stamatouli AM, Inzucchi SE. Implications of the EMPA-REG trial for clinical care and research. *Curr Diab Rep.* 2016;16(12):131.

38. Wanner C, Inzucchi SE, Lachin JM, et al. Empagliflozin and progression of kidney disease in type 2 diabetes. *N Engl J Med.* 2016;375(4):323–334.

39. Scranton R, Cincotta A. Bromocriptine–unique formulation of a dopamine agonist for the treatment of type 2 diabetes. *Expert Opin Pharmacother.* 2010;11(2):269–279.

40. Defronzo RA. Bromocriptine: a sympatholytic, d2-dopamine agonist for the treatment of type 2 diabetes. *Diabetes Care.* 2011;34(4):789–794.

41. Liang W, Gao L, Li N, et al. Efficacy and safety of bromocriptine-QR in type 2 diabetes: a systematic review and meta-analysis. *Horm Metab Res.* 2015;47(11):805–812.

42. Gaziano JM, Cincotta AH, O'Connor CM, et al. Randomized clinical trial of quick-release bromocriptine among patients with type 2 diabetes on overall safety and cardiovascular outcomes. *Diabetes Care.* 2010;33(7):1503–1508.

43. Inzucchi SE. Personalizing glucose-lowering therapy in patients with type 2 diabetes and cardiovascular disease. *Endocrinol Metab Clin North Am.* 2018;47(1):137–152.

44. Qaseem A, Barry MJ, Humphrey LL, Forciea MA. Clinical Guidelines Committee of the American College of P. Oral pharmacologic treatment of type 2 diabetes mellitus: a clinical Practice Guideline update from the American College of Physicians. *Ann Intern Med.* 2017;166(4):279–290.

45. Aronoff S, Rosenblatt S, Braithwaite S, Egan JW, Mathisen AL, Schneider RL. Pioglitazone hydrochloride monotherapy improves glycemic control in the treatment of patients with type 2 diabetes: a 6-month randomized placebo-controlled dose-response study. The Pioglitazone 001 Study Group. *Diab Care.* 2000;23(11):1605–1611.

46. Lebovitz HE, Dole JF, Patwardhan R, Rappaport EB, Freed MI. Rosiglitazone Clinical Trials Study G. Rosiglitazone monotherapy is effective in patients with type 2 diabetes. *J Clin Endocrinol Metab.* 2001;86(1):280–288.

47. Inzucchi SE, Bergenstal RM, Buse JB, et al. Management of hyperglycemia in type 2 diabetes, 2015: a patient-centered approach: update to a position statement of the American Diabetes Association and the European Association for the Study of Diabetes. *Diabetes Care.* 2015;38(1):140–149.

48. Lupsa BC, Inzucchi SE. Diabetes medications and cardiovascular disease: at long last progress. *Curr Opin Endocrinol Diab Obes.* 2018;25(2):87–93.

49. Bennett WL, Wilson LM, Bolen S, et al. *Oral Diabetes Medications for Adults with Type 2 Diabetes: An Update. Rockville (MD);* 2011.

50. Hirst JA, Farmer AJ, Dyar A, Lung TW, Stevens RJ. Estimating the effect of sulfonylurea on HbA1c in diabetes: a systematic review and meta-analysis. *Diabetologia.* 2013;56(5):973–984.

51. Holman RR, Paul SK, Bethel MA, Matthews DR, Neil HA. 10-year follow-up of intensive glucose control in type 2 diabetes. *N Engl J Med.* 2008;359(15):1577–1589.

CHAPTER 13

Bariatric Surgery and Adolescent Type 2 Diabetes

AMY S. SHAH, MD, MS • THOMAS INGE, MD, PHD

The incidence and prevalence of type 2 diabetes (T2D) with onset in adolescence to rise.[1-4] Recent data from The SEARCH for Diabetes in Youth Study estimate that >20,000 youth currently have T2D[2] but by 2050 this rate is expected to quadruple.[5] Similar findings have been seen across the globe in the UK, Japan, and India, where T2D is diagnosed twice as often as type 1 diabetes (T1D) among adolescents.[6-8]

Although the progression to develop T2D in adults occurs over years to decades,[9] T2D in youth has a more rapid onset and higher therapeutic failure rates[10-12] placing adolescents at risk for complications by the age of 30.[13-18] Data from the Treatment Options for Type 2 Diabetes in Adolescents and Youth (TODAY) clinical trial found that dyslipidemia, hypertension, and microalbuminuria are present early among youth with T2D and progress rapidly overtime.[3,19] At baseline, the midadolescent TODAY cohort ($n = 704$) was already severely obese.[3] In just 4 years and despite medical treatment, body mass index increased,[19] rates of hypertension and microalbuminuria tripled, dyslipidemia doubled,[20,21] and glycemic control worsened.[19] Data from a large cohort of T2D adolescents in Cincinnati, Ohio also demonstrate youth with T2D are at risk for early cardiovascular disease.[22-25] At a mean age of 18 years and mean duration of diabetes of 3.5 years, youth with T2D had higher left ventricular mass,[22] worse diastolic function,[22] higher intima media thickening in the carotid artery,[25] and greater peripheral vascular stiffness[24] compared to their obese and lean peers. A Canadian registry also found that complications including dialysis, blindness, and amputation can occur within 10 years of diagnosis of T2D in adolescents. Youth with T2D are also six times more likely to develop vascular disease (compared to age similar controls without T2D).[26] Finally, nephropathy, neuropathy, retinopathy, and cardiovascular death are all higher in adolescents with T2D compared to T1D despite less severe hyperglycemia, virtually no hypoglycemia, and relatively short disease duration.[13-18] Collectively, these findings point to an accelerated risk to develop target organ damage in youth with T2D.[27]

The cornerstone of T2D treatment in adolescence is lifestyle interventions to reduce body weight. However, evidence shows that this approach is unsuccessful in the majority of patients with most adolescents requiring adjunctive pharmacological therapy with metformin and/or subcutaneous insulin.[29,30] The TODAY multicenter randomized controlled trial carefully examined pharmacological failure in children and adolescents with new-onset T2D. The trial defined treatment failure as a hemoglobin A1c of >8% for 6 months or metabolic decompensation requiring insulin therapy.[28] Regardless of therapy, treatment failure was high in all three arms of the trial with 52%, 39%, and 47% of participants failing metformin alone, metformin plus rosiglitazone, and metformin plus lifestyle intervention, respectively, with an average time to failure of 11 months.[19]

Thus, additional therapies to treat adolescent-onset T2D are essential. There is a robust scientific basis demonstrating the effectiveness of bariatric surgery to treat T2D in adult patients. In fact, bariatric surgery is now formally considered not just a weight loss therapy but also a formal treatment of T2D by consensus of dozens of medical and surgical organizations internationally.[29] Although bariatric surgery is not yet standard of care for adolescents, studies in adolescents show bariatric surgery has beneficial effects on T2D outcomes and comorbidities. Here, we will review the common weight loss procedures that have been performed in adolescents, discuss the impact of surgery on T2D and other comorbidities, and discuss the risks of these procedures.

BARIATRIC SURGERY PROCEDURES

Between 2004 and 2011, nearly 950 adolescent bariatric surgery cases per year were performed. From 2004 to 2009, the predominant bariatric procedures

Pediatric Type II Diabetes. https://doi.org/10.1016/B978-0-323-55138-0.00013-9

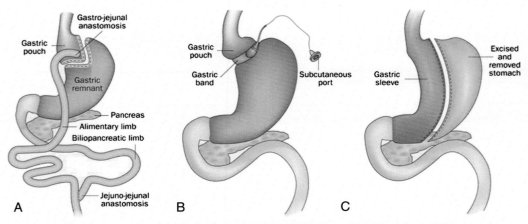

FIG. 13.1 The three most commonly performed bariatric surgery procedures. **(A)** The adjustable gastric band is placed laparoscopically around the upper stomach to restrict the transit of ingested food. **(B)** Laparoscopic sleeve gastrectomy involves separation of the greater curvature from the omentum and splenic attachments. **(C)** Roux-en-Y gastric bypass involves the rearrangement of the alimentary canal, such that ingested food bypasses most of the stomach, all of the duodenum, and a portion of the proximal jejunum. (This figure was originally created and published by Nature Publishing Group © Miras AD, le Roux CW. *Nat Rev Gastroenterol Hepatol*. 2013;10:575–584.)

in adolescents were Roux-en-Y gastric bypass (RYGB) and adjustable gastric banding (AGB) accounting for nearly 86% of all cases. Recent data from 2014 show a shift in the types of procedures performed in adolescents with vertical sleeve gastrectomy (VSG) now accounting for >80% of adolescent cases and together RYGB and AGB being performed <20% of the time (unpublished data). Although these prevalence data provide procedures preferences, there is no clear consensus about which bariatric procedure is most appropriate for adolescents. Each procedure shown in Fig. 13.1 has its advantages and disadvantages along with unique risks.

ADJUSTABLE GASTRIC BAND

The AGB is a purely restrictive procedure in which a rigid, prosthetic band with an inner adjustable balloon is placed laparoscopically around the proximal stomach, usually 1–2 cm below the gastroesophageal junction, thus limiting the volume of food that can be ingested. The balloon within the band inflates with saline using a needle via a subcutaneous port anchored to the fascia of the rectus abdominis muscle to achieve a variable degree of restriction.[30,31] Benefits of this procedure include a lack of staple lines, potential reversibility, and fewer nutritional deficits than the malabsorptive procedures. Complications

include tube leaks, band migration, and erosion of the band into the stomach. Important for the long-term success of the operation, patients are required to follow-up at regular intervals for band adjustment and lifestyle/nutritional counseling. Finally, there is no FDA approval for use of the device in adolescents younger than 18 years of age.

VERTICAL SLEEVE GASTRECTOMY

VSG involves separation of the greater curvature of the stomach from the omentum and splenic attachments and the excision of approximately 75% of the stomach using a stapling device. The excision extends from approximately 5 cm proximal to the pylorus to the angle of His, leaving a narrow remnant stomach based on the lesser curve of the stomach.[31] The benefits of this procedure include the lack of a foreign body, no need for the frequent adjustments as with the AGB and fewer nutritional risks than seen in other malabsorptive procedures. However, leakage from the suture line and stenosis are potential complications.[30,32] Although originally introduced as a first stage procedure that would ultimately entail an additional more definitive bypass type of procedure, the operation appears to be a definitive bariatric operation for most who have undergone the procedure.

ROUX-EN-Y GASTRIC BYPASS

RYGB has been widely adopted in the treatment of severe obesity in the adult population since the 1960s and was first reported for the treatment of severe adolescent obesity as early as the 1970s.[33] It has been described as a combination of a restrictive and malabsorptive procedure. However, more recent investigations in human and animal models suggest that the most important effects of the operation on weight regulation involve physiologic alterations in postprandial gut hormone secretion (affecting appetite and satiety), energy expenditure, macronutrient preference, microbiota, bile acids, and micronutrient and mineral malabsorption.[34] RYGB involves the creation of a small (<30 mL) proximal gastric pouch that is divided and separated from the distal stomach then anastomosed to a Roux limb of small bowel 75–150 cm in length.[35] The benefits of RYGB include a proven ability to induce long-term weight loss and to decrease comorbid disease.[36] However, the procedure is irreversible, causes significant change to the normal gut orientation, and carries a very real risk of micronutrient deficiency long term.

In 2013, a systematic review and metaanalysis comparing the degree of weight loss in adolescents from three different surgeries was published.[37] In total, 637 adolescents undergoing AGB, VSG, and RYGB from 23 studies were included. Mean preoperative BMI for all adolescents ranged from 38.5 to 60.2 kg/m^2 (mean 47.9 kg/m^2). At 1 year, the mean BMI loss was −13.5 kg/m^2 (95% confidence interval −14.1 to −11.9). When examined by procedure type, weight loss was greatest for RYGB (−17.2 kg/m^2, 95% CI −20.1, −14.3), smallest for AGB (−10.5 kg/m^2, 95% CI −11.8, −9.1) and intermediate for VSG (−14.5 kg/m^2, 95% CI −17.3, −11.7). Complication rates were lower for VSG compared to RYGB but were inconsistently reported across adolescent studies.

TYPE 2 DIABETES

Not surprisingly, the weight loss achieved with bariatric surgery is superior to nonsurgical treatments.[38] There is also a potent antidiabetes effect observed with VSG and RYGB which often precedes weight loss[39-45] and persists beyond the perioperative caloric restriction suggesting an independent effect of the surgery on glucose metabolism.[44] Several mechanisms for this weight independent effect have been proposed and may involve improved satiety,[46-48] decreased preference for calorically dense foods,[49,50] or alterations in the gut microbiome,[51-53] bile acid

secretion,[54] and gut hormone production.[55,56] Gastrointestinal hormones including glucose-dependent insulinotropic polypeptide (GIP), glucagon-like peptide (GLP-1), peptide YY (P-YY), ghrelin, and others have been implicated. GIP and GLP-1, specifically, are incretins that decrease blood sugar levels in a glucose-dependent manner by enhancing pancreatic insulin secretin. Postprandial GLP-1 and GIP are increased following bariatric surgery.[57,58] Proposed mechanisms for the gut hormone increases include the passage of more intact nutrients to the ileum through anatomical changes, increased intestinal or bypassing the upper small intestine.[59]

Some of the most robust data examining T2D outcomes after surgery come from the adult Swedish Obese Subjects study. This study found that not only bariatric surgery is superior to lifestyle intervention to reduce the incidence of T2D in obese adults (28.4 compared to 6.8 cases per 1000 patients over 15 years[60]) but also the surgery induces a high rate of T2D remission compared to no surgery (remission of 30% vs. 6.5%[61]). Importantly, the risk of developing microvascular complications from diabetes in their surgical group was approximately one-half of that observed in the control group that did not have surgery.[62]

Similar findings have been published in the 3-year longitudinal study, the STAMPEDE trial,[63] where 40% of adults undergoing RYGB experienced T2D remission as compared with no patients treated with lifestyle intervention alone. The STAMPEDE trial also compared rates of T2D remission by surgery type. T2D remission was observed in 38% of RYGB patients versus 24% of VSG patients.[64] However, the 5-year follow-up to this study showed comparable rates of diabetes remission after both surgeries (29% and 23% of patients, respectively, at 5 years) versus only 5% of patients treated with intensive medical therapy.[65] Though some studies do document slow and steady recurrence of diabetes in surgical patients who initially experience T2D remission, the rates of diabetes do not approach the levels in nonoperated control subjects.[66] Higher rates of T2D relapse in adults have been associated with weight regain, longer duration of diabetes, and insulin use prior to surgery.[66,67]

The effects of bariatric surgery on T2D remission in adolescents have been less studied but initial are promising with remission rates that appear to be higher than those in adults.[68-72] Currently, surgery is recommended for adolescents (age <18 years) who meet clinical criteria for T2D and have severe obesity (defined as an absolute body mass index ≥35 kg/m^2

or a BMI ≥120% of the 95th percentile for age and gender).[36]

Messiah et al. analyzed adolescent T2D outcomes from the Bariatric Outcomes Longitudinal Database, a large-scale surgical quality assurance project.[73] In this analysis, 65 adolescents (15% of all adolescent patients) with T2D underwent AGB, while another 67 (15% of all adolescent patients) underwent gastric bypass. Although the precise definition of T2D remission was not provided, improvement in T2D was reported in 59% of ABG participants and 79% of gastric bypass patients.[73]

Another retrospective cohort study from five adolescent centers reported 1 year outcomes of 11 adolescents with T2D undergoing gastric bypass.[71] At 1-year follow-up, a 33% decrease in BMI was observed. Remission of T2D defined as a fasting glucose <126 mg/dL without medications for T2D was observed for 8 of the 9 evaluable subjects (89% remission), while 2 of 11 (18%) had insufficient data for characterization of diabetes status.

The Teen-LABS study enrolled 23 adolescents with T2D who underwent RYGB (14% of all gastric bypass participants).[74] Of these, there was insufficient data available to classify a diabetes treatment response in five participants. In the remaining 18 participants, remission of T2D (hemoglobin A1c<6.5% without medications) was observed in 17 (94% remission, 95% confidence interval 84%–100%) after 3 years of follow-up. Additionally, no incident cases of T2D were observed over 3 years in the 153 severely obese adolescents undergoing surgery who did not have T2D at baseline. An additional six patients with T2D in the Teen-LABS study underwent VSG. Sufficient data from two of these six were available to assess diabetes response and both were in remission at 3 years. The statistically modeled results, taking into account all available data on these patients between baseline and 3 years, resulted in a modeled remission rate of 90% for those with T2D.

Recently, 3 year outcomes of a larger adolescent cohort ($n = 52$) undergoing VSG were published.[75] In this analysis, all 52 patients were represented in the 3-year outcome. Remission of T2D (fasting glucose < 7 mmol/L, hemoglobin A1c <6.5% and without medications for T2D) was observed in 46/52 (88%) and glucose improvement (decrease in glucose or hemoglobin A1c and decreased T2D medication use) was observed in the remaining six patients (12%).

Studies of adults using comparable definitions of diabetes response have estimated remission rates of approximately 40%–70%. Thus, the T2D remission rates of 88%–90% in adolescents with T2D undergoing RYGB and VSG appear to indicate similar if not greater metabolic effectiveness of surgery when used in adolescents compared to similar operations in adults with T2D. It is unclear why adolescents may have better treatment responses compared to adults but this observation may be related to younger age at surgery, shorter duration of T2D, less medications at baseline, or greater β-cell resilience in youth.[76,77]

CARDIOVASCULAR RISK

Cardiovascular disease is an important T2D-related comorbidity.[78] Bariatric surgery in adults mitigates cardiovascular disease by improving 10-year Framingham cardiovascular risk scores[79,80] and New York Heart Association functional status.[81] This may be related to potent increases in high-density lipoprotein levels, reduction in atherogenic dyslipidemia, and reduction in hypertension following bariatric surgery in adults[82,83] and adolescents[68,72] with comparable outcomes after VSG and RYGB.[84,85] In adolescents, reductions in total cholesterol, LDL, and triglyceride levels with increases in HDL cholesterol levels were observed at 1 year[71,86] that persisted beyond 5 years. Dyslipidemia resolved in 2/3 of patients undergoing bariatric surgery.[87,88] Similarly, reductions in both systolic and diastolic blood pressure have been documented 1 year after RYGB in adolescents[71,86] that persisted after 5 years.[72]

It is not yet clear whether adolescent bariatric surgery influences long-term cardiovascular risk but preliminary data are promising.[89] For example, in adolescents, left ventricular mass as well as thickness of the posterior wall and septum declines after RYGB[89] leading to improved diastolic function. Further study is essential to understand whether younger age at time of surgery may confer benefit in terms of cardiovascular risk reduction.

MICROVASCULAR DISEASE

It appears that the antidiabetic effect of bariatric surgery may also slow or reverse diabetes-related renal damage as indicated by a decrease in the presence of albuminuria[90–93] and improved serum creatinine levels.[92,94] In adolescents, 19 of 22 patients followed 3 years after RYGB or VSG had remission of abnormal kidney function[68] suggesting surgery in adolescents may improve the risk for diabetic nephropathy. Retinopathy is another microvascular complication of diabetes that can have devastating consequences on quality of life due to potential for reduced vision and/or blindness. Both RYGB and VSG appear to reduce incidence of diabetic retinopathy.[95–97] However, risk for new-onset diabetic retinopathy is not eliminated by surgery and progression of existing diabetic retinopathy can occur.[95,96,98] Thus, further work is essential to understand the impact of surgery on retinopathy outcomes. Less is known about the effect of bariatric surgery on risk for diabetic neuropathy, but a survey of patients after RYGB has indicated stability and/or improvement of diabetic neuropathy after RYGB.[99] This has not been studied systematically.

POLYCYSTIC OVARIAN SYNDROME AND FERTILITY

The prevalence of polycystic ovarian syndrome (PCOS) as well as associated menstrual irregularity, hirsutism, and infertility are improved by bariatric surgery including VSG, RYGB, and AGB.[100] A recent metaanalysis indicates that bariatric surgery reduced rates of PCOS from 45.6% preoperatively to only 7.1% postoperatively.[100] Infertility rates also improve dramatically in women after bariatric surgery.[101] Among adolescents after RYGB, pregnancy rates are higher than expected for this age group[102] possibly due to a combination of physiologic and psychosocial changes after surgery.

NONALCOHOLIC FATTY LIVER DISEASE

Nonalcoholic fatty liver disease (NAFLD) has been documented in up to 2/3 of individuals with T2D.[103] The key features in the pathogenesis of NAFLD are insulin resistance and dyslipidemia leading to excessive triglyceride deposition in the hepatocytes.[104] NAFLD is a continuum of disease ranging from hepatic steatosis alone to nonalcoholic steatohepatitis (NASH) to the most severe end of the spectrum with fibrosis and cirrhosis.[105] Treatment for NAFLD is limited to weight loss and occasionally vitamin E, but there are no established guidelines for optimal medical or dietary interventions specifically targeting NALFD. Manco et al. have published the only controlled trial of bariatric surgery for NASH in adolescents to date. Liver histology was examined prospectively before and 6 and 12 months after VSG ($n=20$) and lifestyle intervention ($n=54$). Reversal of NASH was seen in all patients who underwent surgery with no improvement in those who did not undergo surgery.

POTENTIAL COMPLICATIONS

Although remission rates of T2D and its associated comorbidities appear high, there are clear risks from surgery, including surgical and nutritional complications that need to be considered. Surgical outcomes from a single children's hospital that included 77 consecutive gastric bypass procedures found intraoperative complications in 3% of youth, perioperative complications (defined as a complication within 30 days) in 22%, and later complications (between 31 and 90 days) in 13%.[106] The most common postoperative complications included gastrojejunal anastomotic stricture (17%), reoperation (13%), leak (7%), and dehydration (7%).[106] Multicenter prospective complication data over 3 years were reported in the Teen-LABS study in 161 patients undergoing gastric bypass and 67 patients undergoing vertical sleeve gastrectomy.[74] Over 3 years, 13% ($n=30$; 14% of gastric bypass patients and 10% of vertical sleeve gastrectomy participants) of adolescents required 47 additional intraabdominal procedures, most commonly cholecystectomy. Serious complications such as anastomotic leakage were infrequently observed after each type of procedure. Upper endoscopic procedures (including stricture dilations) were experienced by 15% and 7% of gastric bypass and vertical sleeve gastrectomy participants, respectively.

Nutritional deficiencies including vitamin B12, thiamine, and vitamin D deficiency are also a potential short- and long-term complication of bariatric surgery.[74] The Teen-LABS study showed 37% of patients were vitamin D deficient at baseline and 43% of gastric bypass and vertical sleeve gastrectomy patients remained deficient at 3 years. Vitamin B12 deficiency increased from 1% at baseline to 8% at 3 years ($P=.005$). Additionally, low ferritin levels were seen in 57% 3 years after surgery compared to 5% of patients at baseline ($P<.001$).[74] A comprehensive meta-analysis describing surgical and nutritional complications following all bariatric procedures in obese children and adolescents has been published.[37] Complications for adolescents with T2D have not been analyzed separately.

CONCLUSIONS

Accumulating evidence suggests that T2D in adolescents is more aggressive than T2D in adults. T2D in youth results in early multisystem target organ damage over time, likely the combined result of hyperglycemia, hypertension, and dyslipidemia among other risk factors. Data from clinical studies on bariatric surgery in adolescents demonstrate substantial improvement in T2D as well as its associated complications including dyslipidemia, hypertension, and kidney disease though a risk for complications exists. Although further research is still essential to determine the optimal timing and type of surgery for adolescents with T2D, the current data support the recommendations for bariatric surgical management of appropriately selected severely obese adolescents with T2D.[36,107]

REFERENCES

1. Pinhas-Hamiel O, Zeitler P. The global spread of type 2 diabetes mellitus in children and adolescents. *J Pediatr.* 2005;146:693–700.
2. Dabelea D, Mayer-Davis EJ, Saydah S, et al. Prevalence of type 1 and type 2 diabetes among children and adolescents from 2001 to 2009. *JAMA.* 2014;311:1778–1786.
3. Copeland KC, Zeitler P, Geffner M, et al. Characteristics of adolescents and youth with recent-onset type 2 diabetes: the TODAY cohort at baseline. *J Clin Endocrinol Metab.* 2011;96:159–167.
4. Pinhas-Hamiel O, Dolan LM, Daniels SR, Standiford D, Khoury PR, Zeitler P. Increased incidence of non-insulin-dependent diabetes mellitus among adolescents. *J Pediatr.* 1996;128:608–615.
5. Imperatore G, Boyle JP, Thompson TJ, et al. Projections of type 1 and type 2 diabetes burden in the U.S. population aged <20 years through 2050: dynamic modeling of incidence, mortality, and population growth. *Diabetes Care.* 2012;35:2515–2520.
6. Amutha A, Datta M, Unnikrishnan IR, et al. Clinical profile of diabetes in the young seen between 1992 and 2009 at a specialist diabetes centre in south India. *Prim Care Diabetes.* 2011;5:223–229.
7. Urakami T, Suzuki J, Mugishima H, et al. Screening and treatment of childhood type 1 and type 2 diabetes mellitus in Japan. *Pediatr Endocrinol Rev.* 2012;10(suppl 1):51–61.
8. Ehtisham S, Barrett TG, Shaw NJ. Type 2 diabetes mellitus in UK children–an emerging problem. *Diabet Med.* 2000;17:867–871.
9. Meigs JB, Muller DC, Nathan DM, Blake DR, Andres R. The natural history of progression from normal glucose tolerance to type 2 diabetes in the Baltimore Longitudinal Study of Aging. *Diabetes.* 2003;52:1475–1484.
10. Bacha F, Gungor N, Lee S, Arslanian SA. Progressive deterioration of beta-cell function in obese youth with type 2 diabetes. *Pediatr Diabetes.* 2013;14:106–111.
11. D'Adamo E, Caprio S. Type 2 diabetes in youth: epidemiology and pathophysiology. *Diabetes Care.* 2011;34(suppl 2):S161–S165.
12. Effects of metformin, metformin plus rosiglitazone, and metformin plus lifestyle on insulin sensitivity and beta-cell function in TODAY. *Diabetes Care.* 2013;36:1749–1757.
13. Eppens MC, Craig ME, Cusumano J, et al. Prevalence of diabetes complications in adolescents with type 2 compared with type 1 diabetes. *Diabetes Care.* 2006;29:1300–1306.
14. Maahs DM, Snively BM, Bell RA, et al. Higher prevalence of elevated albumin excretion in youth with type 2 than type 1 diabetes: the SEARCH for Diabetes in Youth study. *Diabetes Care.* 2007;30:2593–2598.
15. Constantino MI, Molyneaux L, Limacher-Gisler F, et al. Long-term complications and mortality in young-onset diabetes: type 2 diabetes is more hazardous and lethal than type 1 diabetes. *Diabetes Care.* 2013;36:3863–3869.
16. Dart AB, Sellers EA, Martens PJ, Rigatto C, Brownell MD, Dean HJ. High burden of kidney disease in youth-onset type 2 diabetes. *Diabetes Care.* 2012;35:1265–1271.
17. Jaiswal M, Lauer A, Martin CL, et al. Peripheral neuropathy in adolescents and young adults with type 1 and type 2 diabetes from the SEARCH for Diabetes in Youth follow-up cohort: a pilot study. *Diabetes Care.* 2013;36:3903–3908.
18. Mayer-Davis EJ, Davis C, Saadine J, et al. Diabetic retinopathy in the SEARCH for diabetes in youth cohort: a pilot study. *Diabetes Med.* 2012;29:1148–1152.
19. Zeitler P, Hirst K, Pyle L, et al. A clinical trial to maintain glycemic control in youth with type 2 diabetes. *N Engl J Med.* 2012;366:2247–2256.
20. Lipid and inflammatory cardiovascular risk worsens over 3 years in youth with type 2 diabetes: the TODAY clinical trial. *Diabetes Care.* 2013;36:1758–1764.
21. Rapid rise in hypertension and nephropathy in youth with type 2 diabetes: the TODAY clinical trial. *Diabetes Care.* 2013;36:1735–1741.
22. Shah AS, Khoury PR, Dolan LM, et al. The effects of obesity and type 2 diabetes mellitus on cardiac structure and function in adolescents and young adults. *Diabetologia.* 2011;54:722–730.
23. Urbina EM, Dolan LM, McCoy CE, Khoury PR, Daniels SR, Kimball TR. Relationship between elevated arterial stiffness and increased left ventricular mass in adolescents and young adults. *J Pediatr.* 2011;158:715–721.
24. Urbina EM, Kimball TR, Khoury PR, Daniels SR, Dolan LM. Increased arterial stiffness is found in adolescents with obesity or obesity-related type 2 diabetes mellitus. *J Hypertens.* 2010;28:1692–1698.
25. Urbina EM, Kimball TR, McCoy CE, Khoury PR, Daniels SR, Dolan LM. Youth with obesity and obesity-related type 2 diabetes mellitus demonstrate abnormalities in carotid structure and function. *Circulation.* 2009;119:2913–2919.
26. Dart AB, Martens PJ, Rigatto C, Brownell MD, Dean HJ, Sellers EA. Earlier onset of complications in youth with type 2 diabetes. *Diabetes Care.* 2014;37:436–443.
27. Maahs DM, Daniels SR, de Ferranti SD, et al. Cardiovascular disease risk factors in youth with diabetes mellitus: a scientific statement from the american heart association. *Circulation.* 2014;130:1532–1558.
28. Zeitler P, Epstein L, Grey M, et al. Treatment options for type 2 diabetes in adolescents and youth: a study of the comparative efficacy of metformin alone or in combination with rosiglitazone or lifestyle intervention in adolescents with type 2 diabetes. *Pediatr Diabetes.* 2007;8:74–87.
29. Rubino F, Nathan DM, Eckel RH, et al. Metabolic Surgery in the Treatment Algorithm for Type 2 Diabetes: a joint statement by International Diabetes Organizations. *Surg Obes Relat Dis.* 2016;12:1144–1162.

30. Hsia DS, Fallon SC, Brandt ML. Adolescent bariatric surgery. *Arch Pediatr Adolesc Med.* 2012;166:757–766.
31. Beamish AJ, Olbers T, Kelly AS, Inge TH. Cardiovascular effects of bariatric surgery. *Nat Rev Cardiol.* 2016;13:730–743.
32. Stroh C, Birk D, Flade-Kuthe R, et al. Results of sleeve gastrectomy-data from a nationwide survey on bariatric surgery in Germany. *Obes Surg.* 2009;19:632–640.
33. Thakkar RK, Michalsky MP. Update on bariatric surgery in adolescence. *Curr Opin Pediatr.* 2015;27:370–376.
34. Evers SS, Sandoval DA, Seeley RJ. The physiology and molecular underpinnings of the effects of bariatric surgery on obesity and diabetes. *Annu Rev Physiol.* 2017;79:313–334.
35. Kumar S, Kelly AS. Review of childhood obesity: from epidemiology, etiology, and comorbidities to clinical assessment and treatment. *Mayo Clin Proc.* 2017;92:251–265.
36. Pratt JS, Lenders CM, Dionne EA, et al. Best practice updates for pediatric/adolescent weight loss surgery. *Obes (Silver Spring).* 2009;17:901–910.
37. Black JA, White B, Viner RM, Simmons RK. Bariatric surgery for obese children and adolescents: a systematic review and meta-analysis. *Obes Rev.* 2013;14:634–644.
38. Lawson ML, Kirk S, Mitchell T, et al. One-year outcomes of Roux-en-Y gastric bypass for morbidly obese adolescents: a multicenter study from the Pediatric Bariatric Study Group. *J Pediatr Surg.* 2006;41:137–143; discussion -43.
39. Wickremesekera K, Miller G, Naotunne TD, Knowles G, Stubbs RS. Loss of insulin resistance after Roux-en-Y gastric bypass surgery: a time course study. *Obes Surg.* 2005;15:474–481.
40. Rizzello M, Abbatini F, Casella G, Alessandri G, Fantini A, Leonetti F, Basso N. Early postoperative insulin-resistance changes after sleeve gastrectomy. *Obes Surg.* 2010;20:50–55.
41. Basso N, Capoccia D, Rizzello M, et al. First-phase insulin secretion, insulin sensitivity, ghrelin, GLP-1, and PYY changes 72 h after sleeve gastrectomy in obese diabetic patients: the gastric hypothesis. *Surg Endosc.* 2011;25(2):444–449.
42. Rubino FL, R'Bibo S, del Genio F, Mazumdar M, McGraw TE. Metabolic surgery: the role of the gastrointestinal tract in diabetes mellitus. *Nat Rev Endocrinol.* 2010;6:102–109.
43. Rubino F, Gagner M, Gentileschi P, et al. The early effect of the Roux-en-Y gastric bypass on hormones involved in body weight regulation and glucose metabolism. *Ann Surg.* 2004;240:236–242.
44. Pories WJ, Swanson MS, MacDonald KG, et al. Who would have thought it? An operation proves to be the most effective therapy for adult-onset diabetes mellitus. *Ann Surg.* 1995;222:339–350; discussion 50–52.
45. Schauer PR, Burguera B, Ikramuddin S, et al. Effect of laparoscopic Roux-en Y gastric bypass on type 2 diabetes mellitus. *Ann Surgery.* 2003;238:467–484; discussion 84–85.
46. Lang T, Hauser R, Buddeberg C, Klaghofer R. Impact of gastric banding on eating behavior and weight. *Obes Surg.* 2002;12:100–107.
47. Ullrich J, Ernst B, Wilms B, Thurnheer M, Schultes B. Roux-en Y gastric bypass surgery reduces hedonic hunger and improves dietary habits in severely obese subjects. *Obes Surg.* 2013;23:50–55.
48. Cushing CC, Benoit SC, Peugh JL, Reiter-Purtill J, Inge TH, Zeller MH. Longitudinal trends in hedonic hunger after Roux-en-Y gastric bypass in adolescents. *Surg Obes Relat Dis.* 2014;10:125–130.
49. Ochner CN, Kwok Y, Conceicao E, et al. Selective reduction in neural responses to high calorie foods following gastric bypass surgery. *Ann Surg.* 2011;253:502–507.
50. Faulconbridge LF, Ruparel K, Loughead J, et al. Changes in neural responsivity to highly palatable foods following roux-en-Y gastric bypass, sleeve gastrectomy, or weight stability: an fMRI study. *Obes (Silver Spring).* 2016;24:1054–1060.
51. Furet JP, Kong LC, Tap J, et al. Differential adaptation of human gut microbiota to bariatric surgery-induced weight loss: links with metabolic and low-grade inflammation markers. *Diabetes.* 2010;59:3049–3057.
52. Zhang H, DiBaise JK, Zuccolo A, et al. Human gut microbiota in obesity and after gastric bypass. *Proc Natl Acad Sci U S A.* 2009;106:2365–2370.
53. Sweeney TE, Morton JM. The human gut microbiome: a review of the effect of obesity and surgically induced weight loss. *JAMA Surg.* 2013;148:563–569.
54. Noel OF, Still CD, Argyropoulos G, Edwards M, Gerhard GS. Bile acids, FXR, and metabolic effects of bariatric surgery. *J Obes.* 2016;2016:4390254.
55. Jorgensen NB, Dirksen C, Bojsen-Moller KN, et al. Exaggerated glucagon-like peptide 1 response is important for improved beta-cell function and glucose tolerance after Roux-en-Y gastric bypass in patients with type 2 diabetes. *Diabetes.* 2013;62:3044–3052.
56. Holst JJ. Postprandial insulin secretion after gastric bypass surgery: the role of glucagon-like peptide 1. *Diabetes.* 2011;60:2203–2205.
57. Tsoli M, Chronaiou A, Kehagias I, Kalfarentzos F, Alexandrides TK. Hormone changes and diabetes resolution after biliopancreatic diversion and laparoscopic sleeve gastrectomy: a comparative prospective study. *Surg Obes Relat Dis.* 2013;9:667–677.
58. Shankar SS, Mixson LA, Chakravarthy M, et al. Metabolic improvements following Roux-en-Y surgery assessed by solid meal test in subjects with short duration type 2 diabetes. *BMC Obes.* 2017;4:10.
59. Dimitriadis GK, Randeva MS, Miras AD. Potential hormone mechanisms of bariatric surgery. *Curr Obes Rep.* 2017;6(3):253–265.
60. Carlsson LM, Peltonen M, Ahlin S, et al. Bariatric surgery and prevention of type 2 diabetes in Swedish obese subjects. *N Engl J Med.* 2012;367:695–704.

61. Sjostrom L. Review of the key results from the Swedish Obese Subjects (SOS) trial - a prospective controlled intervention study of bariatric surgery. *J Intern Med.* 2013;273:219–234.

62. Sjostrom L, Peltonen M, Jacobson P, et al. Association of bariatric surgery with long-term remission of type 2 diabetes and with microvascular and macrovascular complications. *JAMA.* 2014;311:2297–2304.

63. Schauer PR, Bhatt DL, Kirwan JP, et al. Bariatric surgery versus intensive medical therapy for diabetes–3-year outcomes. *N Engl J Med.* 2014;370:2002–2013.

64. Schauer PR, Bhatt DL, Kirwan JP, et al. Bariatric surgery versus intensive medical therapy for diabetes - 5-year outcomes. *N Engl J Med.* 2017;376:641–651.

65. Schauer PR, Bhatt DL, Kirwan JP, et al. Bariatric surgery versus intensive medical therapy for diabetes - 5-year outcomes. *N Engl J Med.* 2017;376:641–651.

66. Arterburn DE, Bogart A, Sherwood NE, et al. A multisite study of long-term remission and relapse of type 2 diabetes mellitus following gastric bypass. *Obes Surg.* 2013;23:93–102.

67. Brethauer SA, Aminian A, Romero-Talamas H, et al. Can diabetes be surgically cured? Long-term metabolic effects of bariatric surgery in obese patients with type 2 diabetes mellitus. *Ann Surg.* 2013;258:628–636; discussion 36–37.

68. Inge TH, Courcoulas AP, Jenkins TM, et al. Weight loss and health status 3 Years after bariatric surgery in adolescents. *N Engl J Med.* 2016;374:113–123.

69. Vilallonga R, Himpens J, van de Vrande S. Long-term (7 years) follow-up of Roux-en-Y gastric bypass on obese adolescent patients (<18 years). *Obes Facts.* 2016;9:91–100.

70. Al-Sabah SK, Almazeedi SM, Dashti SA, Al-Mulla AY, Ali DA, Jumaa TH. The efficacy of laparoscopic sleeve gastrectomy in treating adolescent obesity. *Obes Surg.* 2015;25:50–54.

71. Inge TH, Miyano G, Bean J, et al. Reversal of type 2 diabetes mellitus and improvements in cardiovascular risk factors after surgical weight loss in adolescents. *Pediatrics.* 2009;123:214–222.

72. Inge TH, Jenkins TM, Xanthakos SA, et al. Long-term outcomes of bariatric surgery in adolescents with severe obesity (FABS-5+): a prospective follow-up analysis. *Lancet Diabetes Endocrinol.* 2017;5:165–173.

73. Messiah SE, Lopez-Mitnik G, Winegar D, et al. Changes in weight and co-morbidities among adolescents undergoing bariatric surgery: 1-year results from the Bariatric Outcomes Longitudinal Database. *Surg Obes Relat Dis.* 2013;9:503–513.

74. Inge TH, Courcoulas AP, Jenkins TM, et al. Weight loss and health status 3 Years after bariatric surgery in adolescents. *N Engl J Med.* 2016;374(2):113–123.

75. Alqahtani AR, Elahmedi MO, Al Qahtani A. Co-morbidity resolution in morbidly obese children and adolescents undergoing sleeve gastrectomy. *Surg Obes Relat Dis.* 2014;10:842–850.

76. Dicker D, Yahalom R, Comaneshter DS, Vinker S. Long-term outcomes of three types of bariatric surgery on obesity and type 2 diabetes control and remission. *Obes Surg.* 2016;26:1814–1820.

77. Shah AS, D'Alessio D, Ford-Adams ME, Desai AP, Inge TH. Bariatric surgery: a potential treatment for type 2 diabetes in youth. *Diabetes Care.* 2016;39:934–940.

78. Heron M, Hoyert DL, Murphy SL, Xu J, Kochanek KD, Tejada-Vera B. Deaths: final data for 2006. *Natl Vital Stat Rep.* 2009;57:1–134.

79. Arterburn D, Schauer DP, Wise RE, et al. Change in predicted 10-year cardiovascular risk following laparoscopic Roux-en-Y gastric bypass surgery. *Obes Surg.* 2009;19:184–189.

80. Torquati A, Wright K, Melvin W, Richards W. Effect of gastric bypass operation on Framingham and actual risk of cardiovascular events in class II to III obesity. *J Am Coll Surg.* 2007;204:776–782; discussion 82–83.

81. McCloskey CA, Ramani GV, Mathier MA, et al. Bariatric surgery improves cardiac function in morbidly obese patients with severe cardiomyopathy. *Surg Obes Relat Dis.* 2007;3:503–507.

82. Zlabek JA, Grimm MS, Larson CJ, Mathiason MA, Lambert PJ, Kothari SN. The effect of laparoscopic gastric bypass surgery on dyslipidemia in severely obese patients. *Surg Obes Relat Dis.* 2005;1:537–542.

83. Karamanakos SN, Vagenas K, Kalfarentzos F, Alexandrides TK. Weight loss, appetite suppression, and changes in fasting and postprandial ghrelin and peptide-YY levels after Roux-en-Y gastric bypass and sleeve gastrectomy: a prospective, double blind study. *Ann Surg.* 2008;247:401–407.

84. Benaiges D, Goday A, Ramon JM, Hernandez E, Pera M, Cano JF. Laparoscopic sleeve gastrectomy and laparoscopic gastric bypass are equally effective for reduction of cardiovascular risk in severely obese patients at one year of follow-up. *Surg Obes Relat Dis.* 2011;7(5):575–580.

85. Woelnerhanssen B, Peterli R, Steinert RE, Peters T, Borbely Y, Beglinger C. Effects of postbariatric surgery weight loss on adipokines and metabolic parameters: comparison of laparoscopic Roux-en-Y gastric bypass and laparoscopic sleeve gastrectomy-a prospective randomized trial. *Surg Obes Relat Dis.* 2011;7(5):561–568.

86. Inge TH, Jenkins TM, Zeller M, et al. Baseline BMI is a strong predictor of nadir BMI after adolescent gastric bypass. *J Pediatrics.* 2010;156:103–108.e1.

87. Inge TH, Jenkins TM, Xanthakos SA, et al. Long-term outcomes of bariatric surgery in adolescents with severe obesity (FABS-5+): a prospective follow-up analysis. *Lancet Diabetes Endocrinol.* 2017;5(3):165–173.

88. Inge TH, Courcoulas AP, Jenkins TM, et al. Weight loss and health status 3 Years after bariatric surgery in adolescents. *N Engl J Med.* 2016;374:113–123.

89. Ippisch HM, Inge TH, Daniels SR, et al. Reversibility of cardiac abnormalities in morbidly obese adolescents. *J Am Coll Cardiol.* 2008;51:1342–1348.

90. Heneghan HM, Cetin D, Navaneethan SD, Orzech N, Brethauer SA, Schauer PR. Effects of bariatric surgery on diabetic nephropathy after 5 years of follow-up. *Surg Obes Relat Dis.* 2013;9:7–14.
91. Stephenson DT, Jandeleit-Dahm K, Balkau B, Cohen N. Improvement in albuminuria in patients with type 2 diabetes after laparoscopic adjustable gastric banding. *Diab Vasc Dis Res.* 2013;10:514–519.
92. Friedman AN, Wolfe B. Is bariatric surgery an effective treatment for type II diabetic kidney disease? *Clin J Am Soc Nephrol.* 2016;11:528–535.
93. Upala S, Wijarnpreecha K, Congrete S, Rattanawong P, Sanguankeo A. Bariatric surgery reduces urinary albumin excretion in diabetic nephropathy: a systematic review and meta-analysis. *Surg Obes Relat Dis.* 2016;12:1037–1044.
94. Zakaria AS, Rossetti L, Cristina M, et al. Effects of gastric banding on glucose tolerance, cardiovascular and renal function, and diabetic complications: a 13-year study of the morbidly obese. *Surg Obes Relat Dis.* 2016;12:587–595.
95. Gorman DM, le Roux CW, Docherty NG. The effect of bariatric surgery on diabetic retinopathy: good, bad, or both? *Diabetes Metab J.* 2016;40:354–364.
96. Merlotti C, Ceriani V, Morabito A, Pontiroli AE. Bariatric surgery and diabetic retinopathy: a systematic review and meta-analysis of controlled clinical studies. *Obes Rev.* 2017;18:309–316.
97. Kim YJ, Kim BH, Choi BM, Sun HJ, Lee SJ, Choi KS. Bariatric surgery is associated with less progression of diabetic retinopathy: a systematic review and meta-analysis. *Surg Obes Relat Dis.* 2017;13:352–360.
98. Amin AM, Wharton H, Clarke M, Syed A, Dodson P, Tahrani AA. The impact of bariatric surgery on retinopathy in patients with type 2 diabetes: a retrospective cohort study. *Surg Obes Relat Dis.* 2016;12:606–612.
99. Schauer PR, Burguera B, Ikramuddin S, et al. Effect of laparoscopic Roux-en Y gastric bypass on type 2 diabetes mellitus. *Ann Surg.* 2003;238:467–484; discussion 84–85.
100. Skubleny D, Switzer NJ, Gill RS, et al. The impact of bariatric surgery on polycystic ovary syndrome: a systematic review and meta-analysis. *Obes Surg.* 2016;26:169–176.
101. Milone M, De Placido G, Musella M, et al. Incidence of successful pregnancy after weight loss interventions in infertile women: a systematic review and meta-analysis of the literature. *Obes Surg.* 2016;26:443–451.
102. Roehrig HR, Xanthakos SA, Sweeney J, Zeller MH, Inge TH. Pregnancy after gastric bypass surgery in adolescents. *Obes Surgery.* 2007;17:873–877.
103. Cusi K, Sanyal AJ, Zhang S, et al. Non-alcoholic fatty liver disease (NAFLD) prevalence and its metabolic associations in patients with type 1 diabetes and type 2 diabetes. *Diabetes Obes Metab.* 2017;19(11):1630–1634.
104. Hafeez S, Ahmed MH. Bariatric surgery as potential treatment for nonalcoholic fatty liver disease: a future treatment by choice or by chance? *J Obes.* 2013;2013:839275.
105. Saggin L, Gorza L, Ausoni S, Schiaffino S. Troponin I switching in the developing heart. *J Biol Chem.* 1989;264:16299–16302.
106. Miyano G, Jenkins TM, Xanthakos SA, Garcia VF, Inge TH. Perioperative outcome of laparoscopic Roux-en-Y gastric bypass: a children's hospital experience. *J Pediatr Surg.* 2013;48:2092–2098.
107. Kelly AS, Barlow SE, Rao G, et al. Severe obesity in children and adolescents: identification, associated health risks, and treatment approaches: a scientific statement from the American Heart Association. *Circulation.* 2013;128:1689–1712.

Index

Note: Page numbers followed by "f" indicate figures and "t" indicate tables.

Printed in the United States
By Bookmasters